Undergraduate Topics in Computer Science

'Undergraduate Topics in Computer Science' (UTiCS) delivers high-quality instructional content for undergraduates studying in all areas of computing and information science. From core foundational and theoretical material to final-year topics and applications, UTiCS books take a fresh, concise, and modern approach and are ideal for self-study or for a one- or two-semester course. The texts are all authored by established experts in their fields, reviewed by an international advisory board, and contain numerous examples and problems, many of which include fully worked solutions.

The UTiCS concept relies on high-quality, concise books in softback format, and generally a maximum of 275–300 pages. For undergraduate textbooks that are likely to be longer, more expository, Springer continues to offer the highly regarded Texts in Computer Science series, to which we refer potential authors.

More information about this series at http://www.springer.com/series/7592

Rasmus R. Paulsen •
Thomas B. Moeslund

Introduction to Medical Image Analysis

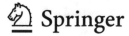 Springer

Rasmus R. Paulsen (ID)
Department for Applied Mathematics
and Computer Science
Technical University of Denmark
Kongens Lyngby, Denmark

Thomas B. Moeslund (ID)
Department of Architecture, Design,
and Media Technology
Aalborg University
Aalborg, Denmark

ISSN 1863-7310   ISSN 2197-1781   (electronic)
Undergraduate Topics in Computer Science
ISBN 978-3-030-39363-2   ISBN 978-3-030-39364-9   (eBook)
https://doi.org/10.1007/978-3-030-39364-9

This Springer imprint is published by the registered company Springer Nature Switzerland AG
The registered company address is: Gewerbestrasse 11, 6330 Cham, Switzerland

Preface

In recent years, there has been a tremendous progress in the use of automatic analysis of images and videos. The field has evolved from being a smaller research area with applications not widely known by the public to have major impact on everyday lives. For example in self-driving cars or face tracking in mobile phones. This rapid increase in the everyday use and the affiliated increase in research impact have also benefitted the life sciences, where medical image analysis plays a major role in modern diagnostics.

The aim of the book is to present the fascinating world of medical image analysis in an easy and interesting way. Compared to many standard books on image analysis, the approach we have chosen is less mathematical and more intuitive. Some of the key algorithms are exemplified in C-code. Please note that the code is neither optimal nor complete and merely serves as an additional input for comprehending the algorithms.

This book is a result of a collaboration between DTU Compute at the Technical University of Denmark (DTU) and the Department of Architecture, Design and Media Technology at Aalborg University, Denmark. It is partly based on the book "Introduction to Video and Image Processing" [5].

For Instructors

We recommend combining the more theoretical exercises found on the homepage with practical exercises where real images are processed. The tools used for practical image analysis is rapidly evolving. Currently, we are using MATLAB for practical exercises and slowly moving to using Python with for example OpenCV or scikit-image. For time critical applications C++ using a good toolkit like for example OpenCV is still preferred. For explorative analysis of images, we often use ImageJ.

Acknowledgements

We would like to thank the following for ideas, figures, and general input: Lars Knudsen, Andreas Møgelmose, Hans Jørgen Andersen, Moritz Störring, David Meredith, Rasmus Larsen, Michael Sass Hansen, Mikkel Stegmann, and Jens Michael Carstensen.

Book Homepage

Updates, exercises and other material with connection to the book can be found on the book homepage: http://mediabook.compute.dtu.dk/.

We hope you will enjoy this book!

Kongens Lyngby, Denmark   Rasmus R. Paulsen
Aalborg, Denmark   Thomas B. Moeslund
January 2020

Contents

Introduction

If we look at the images in Fig. 1.1, we can see two climbers apparently trying to ascend a rock wall. The two persons look content with life and seem to enjoy themselves. We can also estimate their body poses and estimate which muscles are in use. We can detail this description further using adjectives, but we will never *ever* be able to present a textual description, which encapsulates all the details in the images. This fact is normally referred to as "*a picture is worth a thousand words*".

So our eyes and our brain are capable of extracting detailed information far beyond what can be described in text and it is this ability we want to replicate in the "seeing computer". To this end, a camera replaces the eyes and image processing software replaces the human brain. In the medical world, the camera is a more general term that also covers advanced 3D capture devices based on, for example, X-rays. However, most of the methods used to process and analyze these images are the same as the ones used for standard images. The purpose of this book is to present the basics within: cameras, image processing, and image analysis.

Cameras have been around for many years and were initially developed with the purpose of "freezing" a part of the world, for example, to be used in newspapers. For a long time, cameras were analog, meaning that the images were captured on a film. As digital technology matured, the possibility of digital images and image processing became a relevant and necessary science.

Some of the first applications of digital image processing were to improve the quality of the captured images, but as the power of computers grew, so did the number of applications where image and video processing can make a difference. Today image and video processing are used in many diverse applications, such as astronomy (to enhance the quality), medicine (to measure and understand some parameters of the human body, e.g., blood flow in fractured veins or to improve surgery planning using automated analysis of pre-operative 3D images), image compression (to reduce the memory requirement when storing an image), sports (to capture the motion of an athlete in order to understand and improve the performance), rehabilitation (to assess the locomotion abilities), motion pictures (to capture actors' motion in order to

© Springer Nature Switzerland AG 2020
R. R. Paulsen and T. B. Moeslund, *Introduction to Medical Image Analysis*,
Undergraduate Topics in Computer Science,
https://doi.org/10.1007/978-3-030-39364-9_1

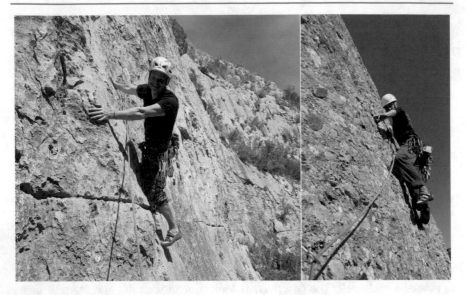

Fig. 1.1 Images containing two climbers on a rock wall. By chance, the two climbers also author books on image analysis

produce special effects based on graphics), surveillance (detect and track individuals and vehicles), production industries (to assess the quality of products), robot control (to detect objects and their pose so a robot can pick them up), TV productions (mixing graphics and live video, e.g., weather forecast), biometrics (to measure some unique parameters of a person), photo editing (improving the quality or adding effects to photographs), and so on.

Many of these applications rely on the same image processing and analysis methods and it is these basic methods which are the focus of this book.

1.1 The Different Flavors of Image Processing

The different image and video processing and analysis methods are often grouped into the categories listed below. There is no unique definition of the different categories and to make matters worse they overlap significantly. Here is one set of definitions:

Image Compression	This is probably the most well-defined category and contains the group of methods used for compressing image and video data.
Image Manipulation	This category covers methods used to edit an image. For example, when rotating or scaling an image, but also when improving the quality by, for example, changing the contrast.

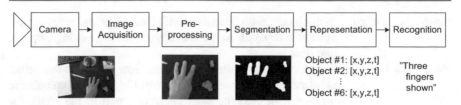

Fig. 1.2 The block diagram provides a general framework for many systems working with images or video

Image Processing	Image processing originates from the more general field of *signal processing* and covers methods used to *segment* the object of interest. Segmentation here refers to methods which in some way enhance the object while suppressing the rest of the image (for example, the edges in an image).
Image Analysis	Here the goal is to analyze the image with the purpose of first finding and second extracting some parameters of the object in the image. For example, finding an object's position and size.
Machine Vision	When applying image processing or image analysis in production industries it is normally referred to as *machine vision* or simply *vision*.
Computer Vision	Humans have *human vision* and similarly a computer has *computer vision*. When talking about computer vision we normally mean advanced algorithms similar to those a human can perform, e.g., face recognition. Normally computer vision also covers all methods where more than one camera is applied.

Even though this book is titled: "Introduction to medical image analysis" it covers methods from several of the above categories in order to provide the reader with a solid foundation for understanding and working with images.

1.2 General Frameworks

Depending on the machines and applications you are working with different general frameworks are relevant. Sometimes not all blocks are included in a particular system, but the framework nevertheless provides a relevant guideline.

In Fig. 1.2 a typical video processing and analysis framework is presented. Underneath each block in the figure, we have illustrated a typical output. The particular outputs are from a gesture-based human-computer-interface system that counts the number of fingers a user is showing in front of the camera.

Below we briefly describe the purpose of the different blocks:

Image Acquisition	In this block, everything to do with the camera and setup of your system is covered, e.g., camera type, camera settings, optics, and light sources.
Pre-processing	This block does something to your image before the actual processing commences, e.g., convert the image from color to gray-scale or crop the most interesting part of the image (as shown in Fig. 1.2).
Segmentation	This is where the information of interest is extracted from the image. Often this block is the "heart" of a system. In the example given in the figure, the information is the fingers. The image below the segmentation block shows that the fingers (together with some noise) have been segmented (indicated by white objects).
Representation	In this block the objects extracted in the segmentation block are represented in a concise manner, e.g., using a few representative numbers as illustrated in the figure.
Recognition	Finally this block examines the information produced by the previous block and classifies each object as being an object of interest or not. In the example in given the figure, this block determines that three finger objects are present and hence output this.

It should be noted that the different blocks might not be as clear-cut defined in reality as the figure suggests. One designer might place a particular method in one block while another designer will place the same method in the previous or following block. Nevertheless, the framework *is* an excellent starting point for any image processing system.

The last two blocks are sometimes replaced by one block called *BLOB Analysis*. This is especially done when the output of the segmentation block is a black and white image as is the case in the figure. In this book, we follow this idea and have therefore merged the descriptions of these two blocks into one—BLOB Analysis.

One typical medical image analysis framework is the analysis of X-ray images. Here, the camera and the acquisition in Fig. 1.2 are replaced with a digital X-ray machine. The recognition block could also be substituted by a *measure* block that measures a physical property of the identified object. It could be a finger length, a cortical bone thickness, or the risk of arthritis.

A more advanced technique is the image acquisition using a computed tomography machine. Here X-ray images are acquired in many different angles around the patient. A 3D volume image is then created by using a set of algorithms normally called *reconstruction*. In this book, we do not cover the 3D image reconstruction topic, but simplifies the framework by just looking at the output from 3D machines as single slice images.

Table 1.1 The organization and topics of the different chapters in this book. # indicates the chapter number

#	Title	Topics
2	Image Acquisition	This chapter describes what light is and how a camera can capture the light and convert it into an image
3	Image Storage	This chapter describes how images can be compressed and stored
4	Point Processing	This chapter presents some of the basic image manipulation methods for understanding and improving the quality of an image. Moreover the chapter presents one of the basic segmentation algorithms
5	Neighborhood Processing	This chapter presents, together with the next chapter, the basic image processing methods, i.e., how to segment or enhance certain features in an image
6	Morphology	Similar to above, but focuses on one particular group of methods for binary images
7	BLOB Analysis	This chapter concerns image analysis, i.e., how to detect, describe, and recognize objects in an image
8	Color Images	This chapter describes what color images are and what they can be used for in terms of segmenting objects
9	Pixel Classification	This chapter describes a statistical method to determine what class of object the pixels in an image represent
10	Geometric Transformation	This chapter deals with another aspect of image manipulation, namely, how to change the geometry within an image, e.g., rotation
11	Registration	In this chapter it is described how two images can be aligned so they are as similar as possible
12	Line and Path Detection	Two different approaches to detect lines and paths in images are described in the chapter

1.3 Deep Learning

In recent years, there has been an explosion in the use of image analysis to solve tasks that were previously considered very hard to solve. A simple example is real-time tracking of human poses, where raw video footage is fed to a computer that finds joint positions of, for example, all players in a football game.

These new applications are largely possible due to new developments within the field of machine learning and in particular the field called *deep learning*. In these years, new papers and applications pushing the limits of what is possible using deep learning are seen every week.

This book is not about deep learning, but to develop and push the limits of modern machine learning, a solid understanding of basic image analysis principles is crucial. Many deep learning networks are based on image convolutions as described in Chap. 5. For pre-processing and data augmentation for deep learning, point processing is often employed (see Chap. 4). The output of a modern segmentation deep learning networks is often post-processed using BLOB analysis as described in Chap. 7.

Therefore, we believe that readers of this book will be better prepared to dive into the rapidly evolving field of machine learning.

1.4 The Chapters in This Book

The chapters in this book are summarized in Table 1.1.

Image Acquisition

2

Before any image processing can commence an image must be captured by a camera and converted into a manageable entity. This is the process known as *image acquisition*. The image acquisition process consists of the steps shown in Fig. 2.1 and can be characterized by three major components; *energy* reflected from the object of interest, an *optical system* which focuses the energy and finally a *sensor* which measures the amount of energy. In Fig. 2.1 the three steps are shown for the case of an ordinary camera with the sun as the energy source. In this chapter, each of these three steps is described in more detail.

2.1 Energy

In order to capture an image, a camera requires some sort of measurable energy. The energy of interest in this context is light or more generally *electromagnetic waves*. An electromagnetic (EM) wave can be described as massless entity, a *photon*, whose electric and magnetic fields vary sinusoidally, hence the name wave. The photon belongs to the group of fundamental particles and can be described in three different ways:

- A photon can be described by its energy E, which is measured in electronvolts [eV]
- A photon can be described by its frequency f, which is measured in Hertz [Hz]. A frequency is the number of cycles or wave-tops in one second
- A photon can be described by its wavelength λ, which is measured in meters [m]. A wavelength is the distance between two wave-tops.

© Springer Nature Switzerland AG 2020

R. R. Paulsen and T. B. Moeslund, *Introduction to Medical Image Analysis*,
Undergraduate Topics in Computer Science,
https://doi.org/10.1007/978-3-030-39364-9_2

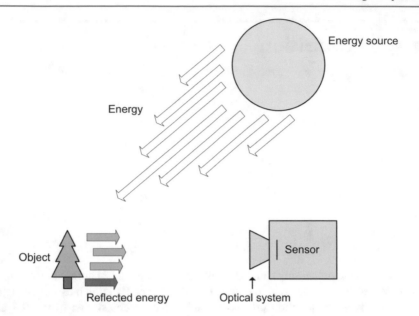

Fig. 2.1 Overview of the typical image acquisition process, with the sun as light source, a tree as object and a digital camera to capture the image. An analog camera would use a film where the digital camera uses a sensor

The three different notations are connected through the speed of light c and Planck's constant h:

$$\lambda = \frac{c}{f} \qquad E = h \cdot f \ \Rightarrow \ E = \frac{h \cdot c}{\lambda} \qquad\qquad (2.1)$$

An EM wave can have different wavelengths (or different energy levels or different frequencies). When we talk about all possible wavelengths we denote this as the *EM spectrum*, see Fig. 2.2.

In order to make the definitions and equations above more understandable, the EM spectrum is often described using the names of the applications where they are used in practice. For example, when you listen to FM-radio the music is transmitted through the air using EM waves around $100 \cdot 10^6 Hz$, hence, this part of the EM spectrum is often denoted "radio". Other well-known applications are also included in Fig. 2.2.

The range from approximately 400–700 nm (nm = nanometer = 10^{-9}) is denoted the visual spectrum. The EM waves within this range are those your eye (and most cameras) can detect. This means that the light from the sun (or a lamp) in principle is the same as the signal used for transmitting TV, radio or for mobile phones, etc. The only difference, in this context, is the fact that the human eye can sense EM waves in this range and not the waves used, for example, radio. Or in other words, if our eyes were sensitive to EM waves with a frequency around $2 \cdot 10^9$ Hz, then your mobile phone would work as a flashlight, and big antennas would be perceived as

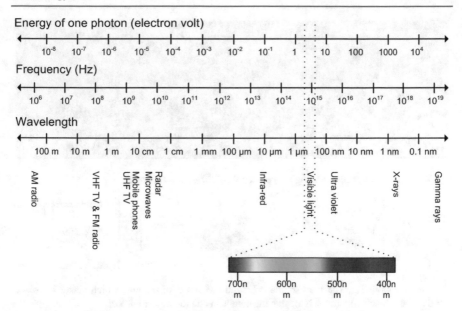

Fig. 2.2 A large part of the electromagnetic spectrum showing the energy of one photon, the frequency, wavelength and typical applications of the different areas of the spectrum

"small suns". Evolution has (of course) not made the human eye sensitive to such frequencies but rather to the frequencies of the waves coming from the sun, hence visible light.

2.1.1 Illumination

To capture an image we need some kind of energy source to illuminate the scene. In Fig. 2.1 the sun acts as the energy source. Most often we apply visual light, but other frequencies can also be applied. For example *x-ray*, which is used to see hard objects within something: bones inside your body or guns in your luggage in airports. Another example is infrared frequencies which are used to see heat, for example, by a rescue helicopter to see people in the dark or by animals hunting at nights. All the concepts, theories, and methods presented throughout this text are general and apply to virtually all frequencies. However, we shall hereafter focus on visual light and denote the energy "light".

If you are processing images captured by others there is nothing much to do about the illumination (although a few methods will be presented in later chapters) which was probably the sun and/or some artificial lighting. When you, however, are in charge of the capturing process yourselves, it is of great importance to carefully think about how the scene should be lit. In fact, for the field of Machine Vision it is a rule-of-thumb that illumination is 2/3 of the entire system design and software only 1/3. To stress this point have a look at Fig. 2.3. The figure shows four images of the

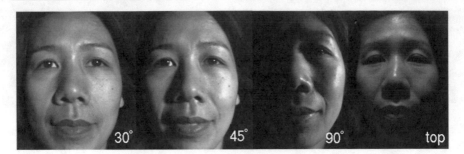

Fig. 2.3 The effect of illuminating a face from four different directions

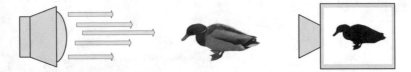

Fig. 2.4 Backlighting. The light source is behind the object of interest, which makes the object stand out as a black silhouette. Note that the details inside the object are lost

same person facing the camera. The only difference between the four images is the direction of the light source (a lamp) when the images were captured!

Another issue regarding the direction of the illumination is that care must be taken when pointing the illumination directly toward the camera. The reason being that this might result in too bright an image or a nonuniform illumination, e.g., a bright circle in the image. If however the outline of the object is the only information of interest, then this way of illumination—denoted backlighting—can be an optimal solution, see Fig. 2.4. Even when the illumination is not directed toward the camera overly bright spots in the image might still occur. These are known as *highlights* and are often a result of a shiny object surface, which reflects most of the illumination (similar to the effect of a mirror). A solution to such problems is often to use some kind of diffuse illumination either in the form of a high number of less-powerful light sources or by illuminating a rough surface which then reflects the light (randomly) toward the object.

Even though this text is about visual light as the energy form, it should be mentioned that infrared illumination is sometimes useful. For example, when tracking the movements of human body parts, e.g., for use in animations in motion pictures, infrared illumination is often applied. The idea is to add infrared reflecting markers to the human body parts, e.g., in the form of small balls. When the scene is illuminated by infrared light, these markers will stand out and can therefore easily be detected by image processing.

2.2 The Optical System

After having illuminated the object of interest, the light reflected from the object now has to be captured by the camera. If a material sensitive to the reflected light is placed close to the object, an image of the object will be captured. However, as illustrated in Fig. 2.5, light from different points on the object will mix—resulting in a useless image. To make matters worse, light from the surroundings will also be captured resulting in even worse results. The solution is, as illustrated in the figure, to place some kind of a barrier between the object of interest and the sensing material. Note also that the image is upside-down. The hardware and software used to capture the image rearranges the image so that you never notice this.

The barrier does more than block out "incorrect" light and in reality the "hole" in the barrier is a complicated optical system. This section describes the basics behind such an optical system. To put it into perspective, the famous space-telescope—the Hubble telescope—basically operates like a camera, i.e., an optical system directs the incoming energy toward a sensor. Imagine how many man-hours were used to design and implement the Hubble telescope. And still, NASA had to send astronauts into space in order to fix the optical system due to an incorrect design. Building optical systems is indeed a complex science! We shall not dwell on all the fine details and the following is therefore not accurate to the last micro-meter, but the description will suffice and be correct for most usages.

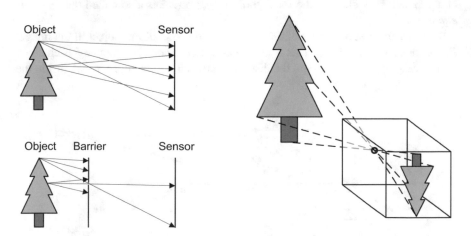

Fig. 2.5 Before introducing a barrier, the rays of light from different points on the tree hit multiple points on the sensor and in some cases even the same points. Introducing a barrier with a small hole significantly reduces these problems

2.2.1　The Lens

One of the main ingredients in the optical system is the lens. A lens is basically
a piece of glass which focuses the incoming light onto the sensor, as illustrated in
Fig. 2.6. A high number of light rays with slightly different incident angles collide
with each point on the object's surface and some of these are reflected toward the
optics. In the figure, three-light rays are illustrated for two different points. All three
rays for a particular point intersect in a point to the right of the lens. Focusing such
rays is exactly the purpose of the lens. This means that an image of the object is
formed to the right of the lens and it is this image the camera captures by placing a
sensor at exactly this position. Note that parallel rays intersect in a point, F, denoted
the *Focal Point*. The distance from the center of the lens, the *optical center O*, to
the plane where all parallel rays intersect is denoted the *Focal Length f*. The line on
which O and F lie is *the optical axis*.

　　Let us define the distance from the object to the lens as, g, and the distance from
the lens to where the rays intersect as, b. It can then be shown that

$$\frac{1}{g} + \frac{1}{b} = \frac{1}{f} \ . \tag{2.2}$$

f and b are typically in the range [1, 100 mm]. This means that when the object is
a few meters away from the camera (lens), then $\frac{1}{g}$ has virtually no effect on the
equation, i.e., $b = f$. What this tells us is that the image inside the camera is formed
at a distance very close to the focal point. Equation 2.2 is also called the *thin lens
equation*.

　　Another interesting aspect of the lens is that the size of the object in the image,
B, increases as f increased. This is known as *optical zoom*. In practice f is changed
by rearranging the optics, e.g., the distance between one or more lenses inside the

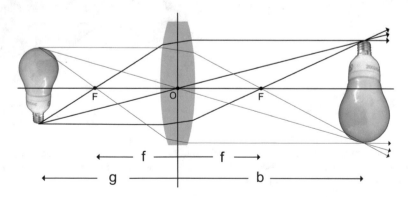

Fig. 2.6 The figure shows how the rays from an object, here a light-bulb, are focused via the lens.
The real light-bulb is to the left and the image formed by the lens is to the right

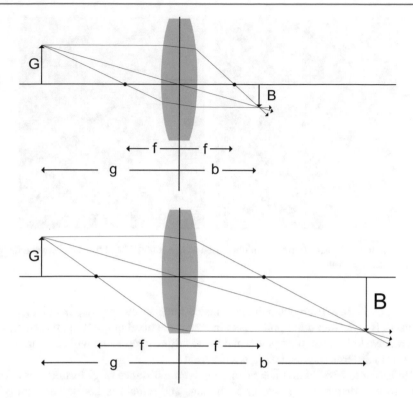

Fig. 2.7 Different focal lengths results in optical zoom

optical system.[1] In Fig. 2.7 we show how optical zoom is achieved by changing the focal length. When looking at Fig. 2.7 it can be shown that

$$\frac{b}{B} = \frac{g}{G} \, , \qquad (2.3)$$

where G is the real height of the object. This can, for example, be used to compute how much a physical object will fill on the imaging sensorchip, when the camera is placed at a given distance away from the object.

Let us assume that we do not have a zoom lens, i.e., f is constant. When we change the distance from the object to the camera (lens), g, Eq. 2.2 shows us that b should also be increased, meaning that the sensor has to be moved slightly further away from the lens since the image will be formed there. In Fig. 2.8 the effect of not changing b is shown. Such an image is said to be *out of focus*. So when you adjust focus on your camera you are in fact changing b until the sensor is located at the position where the image is formed.

The reason for an *unfocused* image is illustrated in Fig. 2.9. The sensor consists of pixels, as will be described in the next section, and each pixel has a certain size.

---

[1]Optical zoom should not be confused with digital zoom, which is done through software.

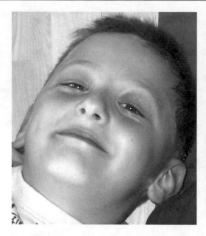 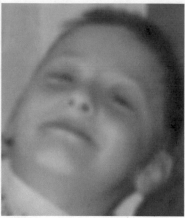

Fig. 2.8 A focused image (left) and an unfocused image (right). The difference between the two images is different values of *b*

As long as the rays from one point stay inside one particular pixel, this pixel will be focused. If rays from other points also intersect the pixel in question, then the pixel will receive light from more points and the resulting pixel value will be a mixture of light from different points, i.e., it is unfocused.

Referring to Fig. 2.9 an object can be moved a distance of g_l further away from the lens or a distance of g_r closer to the lens and remain in focus. The sum of g_l and g_r defines the total range an object can be moved while remaining in focus. This range is denoted as the *depth-of-field*.

A larger depth-of-field can be achieved by increasing the focal length. However, this has the consequence that the area of the world observable to the camera is reduced. The observable area is expressed by the angle V in Fig. 2.10 and denoted the *field-of-view* of the camera. The field-of-view depends, besides the focal length, also on the physical size of the image sensor.

Another parameter influencing the depth-of-field is the *aperture*. The aperture corresponds to the human iris, which controls the amount of light entering the human eye. Similarly, the aperture is a flat circular object with a hole in the center with adjustable radius. The aperture is located in front of the lens and used to control the amount of incoming light. In the extreme case, the aperture only allows rays through the optical center, resulting in an infinite depth-of-field. The downside is that the more light blocked by the aperture, the lower *shutter* speed (explained below) is required in order to ensure enough light to create an image. From this, it follows that objects in motion can result in blurry images.

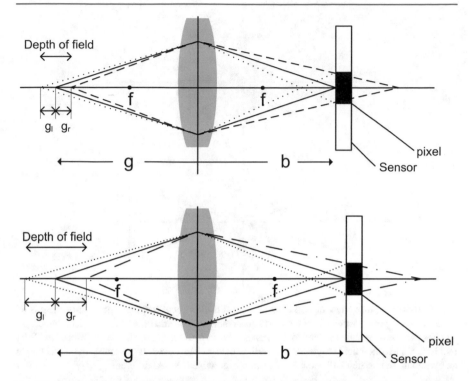

Fig. 2.9 Depth-of-field for two different focal lengths. The solid lines illustrate two light rays from an object (a point) on the optical axis and their paths through the lens and to the sensor where they intersect within the same pixel (illustrated as a black rectangle). The dashed and dotted lines illustrate light rays from two other objects (points) on the optical axis. These objects are characterized by being the most extreme locations where the light rays still enter the same pixel

To sum up, the following interconnected issues must be considered: distance to object, motion of object, zoom, focus, depth-of-field, focal length, shutter, aperture and sensor. In Figs. 2.11 and 2.12 some of these issues are illustrated. With this knowledge, you might be able to appreciate why a professional photographer can capture better images than you can!

2.3 The Imaging Sensor

The light reflected from the object of interest is focused on some optics and now needs to be recorded by the camera. For this purpose, an image sensor is used. An image sensor consists of a 2D array of cells as shown in Fig. 2.13. Each of these cells is denoted a pixel and is capable of measuring the amount of incident light and convert that into a voltage, which in turn is converted into a digital number.

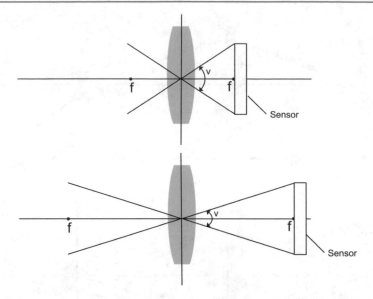

Fig. 2.10 The field-of-view of two cameras with different focal lengths. The field-of-view is an angle, which represents the part of the world observable to the camera. As the focal length increase so does the distance from the lens to the sensor. This in turn results in smaller field-of-view. Note that both a horizontal field-of-view and a vertical field-of-view exist. If the sensor has equal height and width these two fields-of-view are the same, otherwise they are different

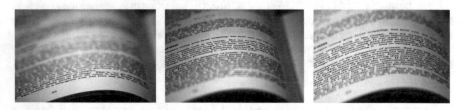

Fig. 2.11 Three different camera settings resulting in three different depth-of-fields

The more incident light the higher the voltage and the higher the digital number. Before a camera can capture an image, all cells are emptied, meaning that no charge is present. When the camera is to capture an image, light is allowed to enter and charges start accumulating in each cell. After a certain amount of time, known as the *exposure time*, and controlled by the *shutter*, the incident light is shut out again. If the exposure time is too low or too high the result is an underexposed or overexposed image, respectively, see Fig. 2.14.

Furthermore, if the object of interest is in motion the exposure time in general needs to be low in order to avoid *motion blur*, where light from a certain point on the object will be spread out over more cells.

The accumulated charges are converted into digital form using an *analog-to-digital converter*. This process takes the continuous world outside the camera and

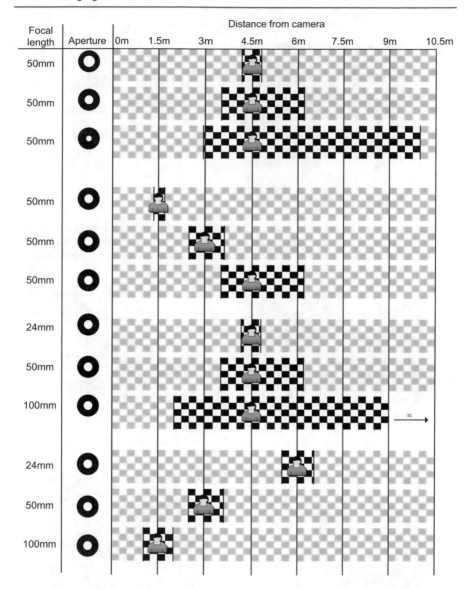

Fig. 2.12 Examples of how different settings for focal length, aperture, and distance to object result in different depth-of-fields. For a given combination of the three settings, the optics are focused so that the object (person) is in focus. The focused checkers then represent the depth-of-field for that particular setting, i.e., the range in which the object will be in focus. The figure is based on a Canon 400D

Sensor   Single cell

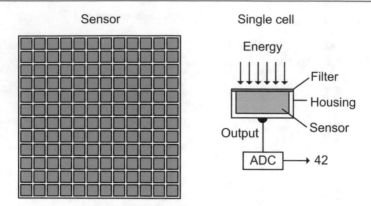

Fig. 2.13 The sensor consists of an array of interconnected cells. Each cell consists of a housing which holds a filter, a sensor, and an output. The filter controls which type of energy is allowed to enter the sensor. The sensor measures the amount of energy as a voltage, which is converted into a digital number through an Analog-To-Digital Converter (ADC)

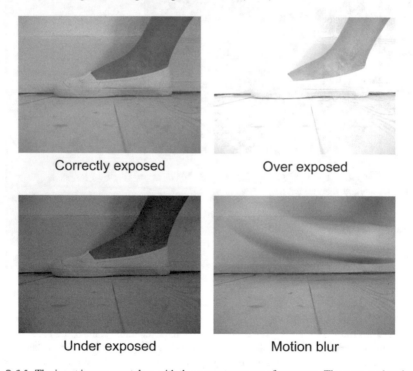

Fig. 2.14 The input image was taken with the correct amount of exposure. The over- and underexposed images are too bright and too dark, respectively, which makes it hard to see details in them. If the object or camera is moved during the exposure time, it produces motion blur as demonstrated in the last image

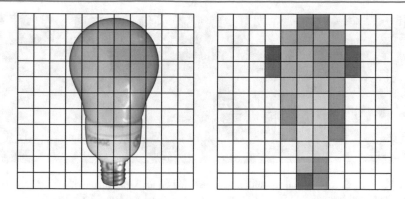

Fig. 2.15 To the left the amount of light which hits each cell is shown. To the right the resulting image of the measured light is shown

converts it into a digital representation, which is required when stored in the computer. Or in other words, this is where the image becomes digital. To fully comprehend the difference, have a look at Fig. 2.15.

To the left we see where the incident light hits the different cells and how many times (the more times the brighter the value). This results in the shape of the object and its intensity. Let us first consider the shape of the object. A cell is sensitive to incident light hitting the cell, but not sensitive to where exactly the light hits the cell. So if the shape should be preserved, the size of the cells should be infinitely small. From this it follows that the image will be infinitely large in both the x- and y-direction. This is not tractable and therefore a cell, of course, has a finite size. This leads to loss of data/precision and this process is termed *spatial quantization*. The effect is the blocky shape of the object in the figure to the right. The number of pixels used to represent an image is also called the *spatial resolution* of the image. A high resolution means that a large number of pixels are used giving fine details in the image. A low resolution means that a relatively low number of pixels is used. Sometimes the words fine and coarse resolution are used. The visual effect of the spatial resolution can be seen in Fig. 2.16. Overall we have a trade-off between memory and shape preservation. It is possible to change the resolution of an image by a process called *image-resampling*. This can be used to create a low-resolution image from a high-resolution image. However, it is normally not possible to create a high-resolution image from a low-resolution image.

A similar situation is present for the representation of the amount of incident light within a cell. The number of photons hitting a cell can be tremendously high requiring an equally high digital number to represent this information. However, since the human eye is not even close to being able to distinguish the exact number of photons, we can quantify the number of photons hitting a cell. Often this quantization results in a representation of one Byte (8 bits), since one byte corresponds to the way memory is organized inside a computer (see Appendix A for an introduction to bits and bytes). In the case of 8-bit quantization, a charge of 0 volt will be quantized to

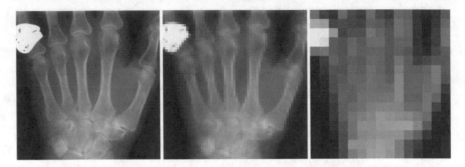

Fig. 2.16 The effect of spatial resolution demonstrated on an X-ray image of a hand (notice the ring). The spatial resolution is from left to right: 256×256, 64×64, and 16×16

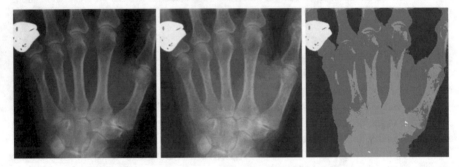

Fig. 2.17 The effect of gray-level resolution demonstrated on an X-ray image of a hand. The gray-level resolution is from left to right: 256, 16, and 4 gray levels

0 and a high charge quantized to 255. Other gray-level quantizations are sometimes used. The effect of changing the gray-level quantization (also called the gray-level resolution) can be seen in Fig. 2.17. With more than 64 gray levels, the visual effect is rather small. Down to 16 gray levels the image will frequently still look realistic, but with a clearly visible quantization effect. Maybe surprisingly the image can still be visually interpreted with only four gray levels. The gray-level resolution is usually specified in number of bits. While, typical gray-level resolutions are 8-, 10-, and 12-bit corresponding to 256, 1024, and 4096 gray levels, 8-bit images are the most common and are the topic of this text (unless otherwise noted).

In the case of an overexposed image, a number of cells might have charges above the maximum measurable charge. These cells are all quantized to 255. There is no way of knowing just how much incident light entered such a cell and we therefore say that the cell is *saturated*. This situation should be avoided by setting the shutter (and/or aperture), and saturated cells should be handled carefully in any image processing system. When a cell is saturated it can affect the neighbor pixels by increasing their changes. This is known as *blooming* and is yet another argument for avoiding saturation.

2.4   Digital Images

To transform the information from the sensor into an image, each cell content is now converted into a pixel value in the range: [0, 255]. Such a value is interpreted as the amount of light hitting a cell during the exposure time. This is denoted the *intensity* of a pixel. It is visualized as a shade of gray denoted a *gray-scale value* or *gray-level value* ranging from black (0) to white (255), see Fig. 2.18.

A gray-scale image (as opposed to a color image, which is the topic of Chap. 8) is a 2D array of pixels (corresponding to the 2D array of cells in Fig. 2.13) each having a number between 0 and 255. A frequent representation of digital images is as matrices or as discrete function values over a rectangular two-dimensional region. An 8-bit gray-scale image is represented as a two-dimensional matrix with M rows and N columns, where each element contains a number between 0 and 255.

2.4.1   Image Coordinate Systems

Unfortunately, several coordinates systems are used for images. In MATLAB where images are considered matrices, pixel coordinates are specified as (row, column) with (1, 1) being placed in the upper left corner. A pixel value will often be written as $v(r, c)$ or just as v, where r is the row number and c is the column number. In some textbooks and systems (x, y) with (0, 0) in the upper left corner is used. Finally, the standard mathematical (x, y) system with (0, 0) in the lower left corner can also be used. The three different systems can be seen in Fig. 2.19.

Systems that uses (0, 0) as origin are said to be 0-based and systems that use (1, 1) are 1-based . An overview of which systems different software packages use can be found in Table 2.1.

In this text, the coordinate 0-based system with (0, 0) in the upper left corner is used, unless otherwise specified. The image is represented as $f(x, y)$, where x is the horizontal position of the pixel and y the vertical position. For the small image in Fig. 2.19 to the left, $f(0, 0) = 23$, $f(3, 1) = 130$, and $f(2, 3) = 7$. It can also be seen that the pixel with value $v = 158$ is placed at $(r, c) = (2, 3)$ in the MATLAB coordinate system, in Photoshop it can be found at $(x, y) = (2, 1)$, and in the mathematical systems at $(x, y) = (2, 2)$.

The conversion between, for example, MATLAB (r, c) and Photoshop coordinates (x, y) is done by $(x, y) = (c - 1, r - 1)$ and $(r, c) = (y + 1, x + 1)$.

So whenever you see a gray-scale image you must remember that what you are actually seeing is a 2D array of numbers as illustrated in Fig. 2.20.

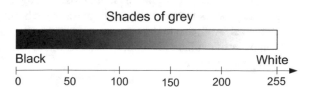

Fig. 2.18 The relationship between the intensity values and the different shades of gray

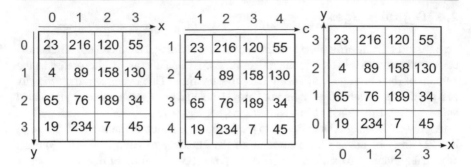

Fig. 2.19 Pixel coordinate systems. The left is the one used by, for example, Photoshop and GIMP. The middle is the standard matrix system used by MATLAB. The right is a standard mathematical coordinate system

Table 2.1 Coordinate systems used by different software packages

Software	Origin	System	Base
MATLAB images	Upper left corner (1, 1) (r, c)		1-based
MATLAB matrices	Upper left corner (1, 1) (r, c)		1-based
C and C++	Upper left corner (0, 0) (x, y)		0-based
VXL (C++)	Upper left corner (0, 0) (x, y)		0-based
Photoshop	Upper left corner (0, 0) (x, y)		0-based
GIMP	Upper left corner (0, 0) (x, y)		0-based
MATLAB plotting	Lower left corner (0, 0) (x, y)		0-based
Many plotting packages	Lower left corner (0, 0) (x, y)		0-based

2.4.2 The Region-of-Interest (ROI)

As digital cameras are sold in larger and larger numbers the development within sensor technology has resulted in many new products including larger and larger numbers of pixels within one sensor. This is normally defined as the size of the image that can be captured by a sensor, i.e., the number of pixels in the vertical direction multiplied by the number of pixels in the horizontal direction. Having a large number of pixels can result in high quality images and has made, for example, digital zoom a reality.

When it comes to image processing, a larger image size is not always a benefit. Unless you are interested in tiny details or require very accurate measurements in the image, you are better off using a smaller sized image. The reason being that when we start to process images we have to process each pixel, i.e., perform some math on each pixel. And, due to the large number of pixels, that quickly adds up to quite a large number of mathematical operations, which in turn means a high computational load on your computer.

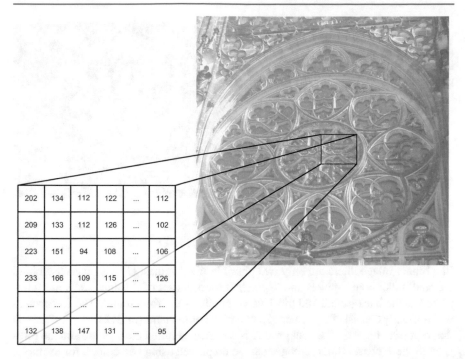

Fig. 2.20 A gray-scale image and part of the image described as a 2D array, where the cells represent pixels and the value in a cell represents the intensity of that pixel

Say you have an image which is 500×500 pixels. That means that you have $500 \cdot 500 = 250.000$ pixels. Now say that you are processing video with 50 images per second. That means that you have to process $50 \cdot 250.000 = 12.500.000$ pixels per second. Say that your algorithm requires 10 mathematical operations per pixel, then in total your computer has to do $10 \cdot 12.500.000 = 125.000.000$ operations per second. That is, quite a number even for today's powerful computers. So when you choose your camera do not make the mistake of thinking that bigger is always better!

Besides picking a camera with a reasonable size you should also consider introducing a *Region-Of-Interest* (ROI). A ROI is simply a region (normally a rectangle) within the image which defines the pixels of interest. Those pixels not included in the region are ignored altogether and less processing is required. An ROI is illustrated in Fig. 2.21.

The ROI can sometimes be defined for a camera, meaning that the camera only captures those pixels within the region, but usually it is something you as a designer define in software. Say that you have put up a camera in your home in order to detect if someone comes through one of the windows while you are on holiday. You could then define an ROI for each window seen in the image and *only* process these pixels. When you start playing around with image processing you will soon realize the need for an ROI.

Fig. 2.21 The rectangle
defines a Region-Of-Interest
(ROI), i.e., this part of the
image is the only one being
processed

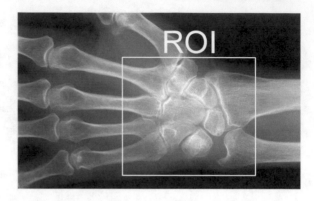

2.4.3 Binary Images

In a binary image, there are only two possible pixel values. Unless otherwise noted
we shall talk about 0-pixels and 1-pixels. Often the set of 0 value pixels are interpreted as the background and the 1 value pixels as the foreground. The foreground
will normally consist of a number of connected components (or BLOBS, see Chap. 7)
that represent objects. The background is sometimes called the 0-phase and the foreground the 1-phase. Binary images can be displayed using two colors, for example,
black and white. Binary images are typically a result of thresholding a gray-level
image as will be described in Sect. 4.4. A binary image can be seen in Fig. 2.22
in the middle, where a computed tomography image of the human brain has been
thresholded so the bone pixels constitute the foreground object.

2.4.4 Label Images

Occasionally, another image representation is used, where the pixel value does not
represent a light intensity but is a number that tells something about the pixel. A
typical example is that the pixel value tells which object the pixel belongs to. If an
image contains a man and a dog, the pixel values could be 0 for pixels belonging to
the background, 1 for pixels that constitute the man, and 2 for dog pixels. Here we
say that the pixels have been labeled with three label values and the image is called
a label image. Label images are typically the result of image segmentation, BLOB
analysis, or pixel classification algorithms. In Fig. 2.22 to the right a label image
can be seen. The different tissue types in the human head have been classified in a
computed tomography image. The labels are visualized using colors, where the gray
pixels are the background, the blue pixels belong to the soft tissue, and the green and
the red pixels belong to two different types of bones.

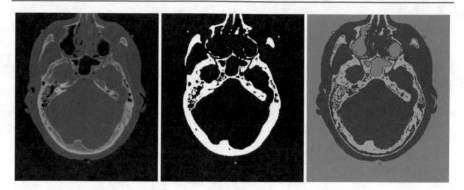

Fig. 2.22 A computed tomography scan of the human head. To the left it is seen as a gray-scale image, in the middle it has been transformed into a binary image, and to the right a label image has been created (gray = background, blue = soft tissue, green and red = bone)

2.4.5 Multi-spectral Images

In a gray-level image there is one measurement (the intensity) per pixel and in color images there are three values per pixel (the red, green, and blue. See Chap. 8). However, it can be useful to measure several intervals of the electromagnetic spectrum individually and in this way assign more than three values per pixel. An example is the addition of near-infrared information to a pixel value. Images containing information captured at multiple spectral wavelengths are called *multi-spectral images* or *multi-channel images*. Images captured by satellites are often multi-spectral. Furthermore, there is extensive research in multi-spectral cameras for diagnostic purposes as, for example, early skin cancer diagnostics.

2.4.6 16-Bit Images

While the human visual system does not need more than 256 different gray levels in an image, a computer can gain more information by having a large pixel value range available. An example is modern medical scanners, where the pixel value does not represent the intensity of incoming light, but an underlying physical measurement. In Computed Tomography (CT) scanners, the pixel value is typically measured in Hounsfield Units (HU) that describe the attenuation of X-rays in the tissue. The Hounsfield unit is defined so a pixel that describes air has a value of 1000 and a pixel describing water has a value of 0. A typical bone pixel will have a value of 400. Obviously, a single byte with 256 different values cannot be used to store these pixel values (see Appendix A for an introduction to bits and bytes). Instead images where each pixel value is stored as two bytes are used. Two bytes equal 16 bits and this type of images is therefore called 16-bit images. A CT scanner normally creates 16-bit images. Certain modern cameras create 10-bit (1024 gray levels) or 12-bit (4096 gray levels) images, where only 10 or 12 of the 16 bits are used, but the pixel values are still stored as two bytes.

Image Storage and Compression

3

When an image is captured, it is normally stored in the memory of the capture device (the camera, for example). However, to store the image permanently it needs to be transferred to another type of storage. This is typically a hard disk or a type of memory card for portable digital cameras. Instead of storing the raw pixel values, it is much better to store the image using an *image file format* and to compress the image information before storing. In this chapter, these processes are described in detail.

As described in Sect. 2.4, an image is normally represented as a 2D array of values or as a matrix. However, when an image is written to a file on, for example, a hard disk it needs to be stored as a one-dimensional sequence of bytes. A matrix can easily be transformed into a sequence by storing each row after each other. A 256-level gray-scale image with 500 rows and 1000 columns will result in a sequence of 500.000 bytes. The image shown in Fig. 3.1 to the left will be represented as a sequence of 16 numbers:

$$23, 23, 23, 55, 55, 89, 89, 55, 55, 55, 158, 34, 34, 34, 34, 34.$$

Some simple image file formats like *Windows BitMap Format* (BMP) uses this representation with an additional *image header*. The header always contains information about the size of the image and if the image is a gray-scale or a color image. In more advanced formats, the header also contains information about the date of capture and camera specific details like shutter time and focal length.

© Springer Nature Switzerland AG 2020

R. R. Paulsen and T. B. Moeslund, *Introduction to Medical Image Analysis*,
Undergraduate Topics in Computer Science,
https://doi.org/10.1007/978-3-030-39364-9_3

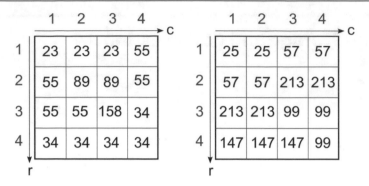

Fig. 3.1 Two gray-scale images

3.1 Lossless Compression and Image Formats

An image written directly to the hard disk takes up the same space (and a little bit more because of the header) as the number of pixels in the image. However, images normally contain regions with very similar colors (or gray-scales) and therefore they can often be *compressed*. Compression means to represent the image data with less bytes than the original data. A simple compression method is Run-Length Encoding (RLE). Here a sequence of values that have the same value (called a *run*) is stored as the count (the number of the values) and the value. The first three pixel in the image in Fig. 3.1 to the left will therefore be stored as 3, 23 instead of 23, 23, 23. The entire image in Fig. 3.1 to the left is stored as

$$3, 23, 2, 55, 2, 89, 3, 55, 1, 158, 5, 34,$$

when it is run-length encoded. The storage is therefore reduced from 16 bytes to 12 bytes. The *compression ratio* is defined as

$$\text{Compression Ratio} = \frac{\text{Uncompressed Size}}{\text{Compressed Size}} . \tag{3.1}$$

In the example above the compression rate is therefore $16 : 12 = 4 : 3 \sim 1.33$, that is, not impressive. However, for larger images it can be effective. The image Fig. 3.1 to the right has the following run-length code: 2, 25, 4, 57, 4, 213, 2, 99, 3, 147, 1, 99 and therefore also the compression ratio of $4 : 3$.

Run-length encoding is a *lossless* compression since the original image data can be computed from the encoded data without any loss. A popular image format that stores images using lossless compression is the *Portable Network Graphics (PNG)* format. However, the compression it uses is much more complex than just run-length encoding and is beyond the scope of this text.

Images that should be analyzed should always be stored using a lossless image format. Some popular image file formats can be seen in Table 3.1.

Table 3.1 A selection of the most popular image formats

Name	File name	Compression	Comment
Joint Photographic Experts Group (JPEG)	myimage.jpg	Lossy	Good for photos Not good for analysis
Portable Network Graphics (PNG)	myimage.png	Lossless	Good for image analysis
Graphics Interchange Format (GIF)	myimage.gif	Lossless	Only 256 colors
Windows BitMap Format (BMP)	myimage.bmp	Lossless	Uncompressed or RLE
Tagged Image File Format (TIFF)	myimage.tif	Lossy or Lossless	Complex format
Digital Imaging and Communications in Medicine (DICOM)	myimage.dcm (not always)	Lossy or Lossless	Very complex format

3.2   Lossy Compression and Image Formats

While run-length encoding can be used for all types of data (sound, signals, and measurements). Dedicated compression algorithms for images also exist. They take advantage of the fact that the human eye has limitations and cannot see all the details in images. A very popular image format Joint Photographic Experts Group (JPEG) is based on computing the *frequencies* in the image and then only storing the frequencies that the human eye can clearly see. It is normally possible to control the amount of data (frequencies) that should be removed when the image is stored. If the compression ratio is too high, it is possible to see *compression artifacts* as shown in Fig. 3.2. With JPEG, the compression artifacts are typically blurred box-like shapes around the sharp edges.

Lossy image compression should generally not be used for images that should be analyzed since the compression artifacts can be mistaken as important information. A

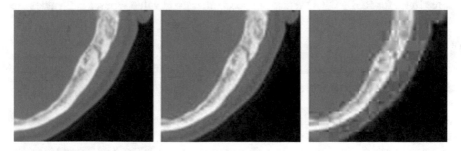

Fig. 3.2 JPEG artifacts. To the left is the original CT skull image. In the middle it is saved with medium JPEG compression and to the right it is saved with very high compression

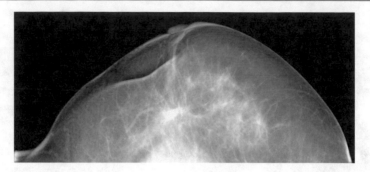

Fig. 3.3 Mammogram. Low dose X-ray image of a human breast. The pattern of tiny bright spots can potentially be used in cancer diagnostics and it is therefore crucial that the micro-structure of the image is not destroyed during image compression

typical example is mammography, where low X-ray images are taken of the human breast. A mammogram can be seen in Fig. 3.3. Breast cancer is detected as, for example, particular patterns and shapes of *microcalcifications* that are seen as tiny bright spots in the image. If lossy compression is used to store this type of images, critical errors may occur in the following diagnosis.

Some complex image formats can store images in both lossy and lossless mode as shown in Table 3.1.

3.3 DICOM

DICOM is an acronym for Digital Imaging and Communications in Medicine (DICOM). As indicated by the title, it is not only a file format but also a *standard* for transmitting images over a network. It is a very complex format that can handle images from almost all medical imaging equipment. The header of the DICOM image typically contains patient information and sometimes also diagnostic information. Compared to the more standard image formats that store one pixel as one byte (or three bytes for RGB) DICOM also supports other pixel value types. Pixel values are often stored as 16-bit (2 bytes).

3.4 Binary Image Compression

Since there are only two possible values in a binary image, specialized compression methods can be used. These methods are based on the simple fact that binary images are fully described just by describing the foreground. The background is easily obtained given the foreground (as all pixels that are not black are white).

Fig. 3.4 Left: numbering of the eight directions. Right: binary image with one black object

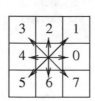

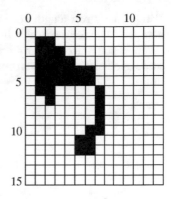

3.4.1 Chain Coding

In chain coding, an object is represented by an arbitrarily chosen starting pixel on the boundary and the sequence of small steps, that is, needed to travel clockwise around the boundary of the object back to the starting pixel. Every step can be in one of eight directions as illustrated in Fig. 3.4 to the left. The numbering of the eight different types of steps is also shown. The binary image in Fig. 3.4 to the right has the chain code:

$$(1, 1)(07770676666564211222344456322222),$$

where $(1, 1)$ is the position of the first pixel of the object. Using the chain code, this binary image can now be described using $2 + 2 + 32 = 36$ numbers. Two describing the height and width of the image, two for the starting pixel position, and 32 for the chain code. The original size of the image is $14 \cdot 16 = 224$ and therefore the compression ratio is $224 : 36 \sim 6.2$.

3.4.2 Run-Length Coding

As described in Sect. 3.1, run-length coding is based on a description of *runs* in a given scan direction. The difference between gray-level run-length coding and binary run-length coding is that we only need to describe the foreground pixel in the binary case. Using horizontal scanning a run is a set of horizontally connected foreground pixels. In a binary run-length code, a run is represented by its row number followed by the column numbers of the first and last pixel. The image in Fig. 3.4 to the right can be described by the run-length code:

$$[1; (1, 2)], [2; (1, 3)], [3; (1, 4)], [4; (1, 6)]$$

$$[5; (1, 6)], [6, (1, 2)(7, 7)], [7; (2, 2)(7, 7)], [8; (7, 7)]$$

$$[9; (7, 7)], [10; (6, 7)], [11; (5, 6)], [12; (5, 6)]$$

Using binary run-length coding, the image information is stored as $2 + 40 = 42$ numbers. Two for the image dimensions and 40 for the run-length code. This gives a compression ratio of $224 : 42 \sim 5.3$. In practical implementations, there are always some overhead, so the given compression ratios should be considered the theoretical limits.

Point Processing

4

Sometimes when people make a movie they lower the overall intensity in order to create a special atmosphere. Some overdo this and the result is that the viewer cannot see anything except darkness. What do you do? You pick up your remote and adjust the level of the light by pushing the brightness button. When doing so you actually perform a special type of image processing known as *point processing*.

Say we have an input image $f(x, y)$ and wish to manipulate it resulting in a different image, denoted the *output image* $g(x, y)$. In the case of changing the brightness in a movie, the input image will be the one stored on the DVD you are watching and the output image will be the one actually shown on the TV screen. Point processing is now defined as an operation which calculates the new value of a pixel in $g(x, y)$ based on the value of the pixel *in the same position* in $f(x, y)$ and some operation. That is, the values of a pixel's neighbors in $f(x, y)$ have no effect whatsoever, hence the name point processing. In the forthcoming chapters, the neighbor pixels *will* play an important role. The principle of point processing is illustrated in Fig. 4.1. In this chapter, some of the most fundamental point processing operations are described.

4.1 Gray-Level Mapping

When manipulating the brightness by your remote you actually change the value of b in the following equation:

$$g(x, y) = f(x, y) + b \tag{4.1}$$

Every time you push the "+" brightness button the value of b is increased and vice versa. The result of increasing b is that a higher and higher value is added to each pixel in the input image and hence it becomes brighter. If $b > 0$ the image becomes brighter and if $b < 0$ the image becomes darker. The effect of changing the brightness is illustrated in Fig. 4.2.

© Springer Nature Switzerland AG 2020

R. R. Paulsen and T. B. Moeslund, *Introduction to Medical Image Analysis*,
Undergraduate Topics in Computer Science,
https://doi.org/10.1007/978-3-030-39364-9_4

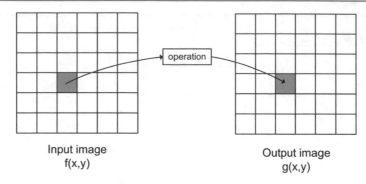

Fig. 4.1 The principle of point processing. A pixel in the input image is processed and the result is stored at the same position in the output image

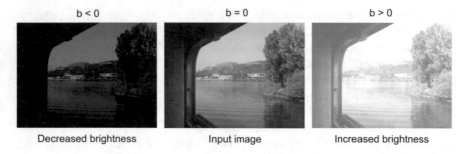

Fig. 4.2 If b in Eq. 4.1 is zero, the resulting image will be equal to the input image. If b is a negative number then the resulting image will have decreased brightness, and if b is a positive number the resulting image will have increased brightness

An often more convenient way of expressing the brightness operation is by means of graphics, see Fig. 4.3. The graph shows how a pixel value in the input image (horizontal axis) maps to a pixel value in the output image (vertical axis). Such a graph is denoted *gray-level mapping*. In the first graph, the mapping does absolutely nothing, i.e., $g(142, 42) = f(142, 42)$. In the next graph, all pixel values are increased ($b > 0$), hence, the image becomes brighter. This results in two things: (i) no pixel will be completely dark in the output and (ii) some pixels will have a value above 255 in the output image. The latter is no good due to the upper limit of an 8-bit image and therefore all pixels above 255 are set equal to 255 as illustrated by the horizontal part of the graph. When $b < 0$ some pixels will have negative values and are therefore set equal to zero in the output as seen in the last graph.

Just like changing the brightness on your TV, you can also change the *contrast*. The contrast of an image is a matter of how different the gray-level values are. If we look at two pixels next to each other with values 112 and 114, then the human eye has difficulties distinguishing them and we will say there is a *low* contrast. On the other hand, if the pixels are 112 and 212, respectively, then we can easily distinguish

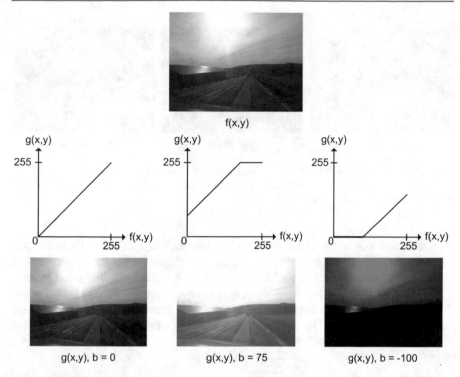

Fig. 4.3 Three examples of gray-level mapping. The top image is the input. The three other images are the result of applying the three gray-level mappings to the input. All three gray-level mappings are based on Eq. 4.1

them and we will say the contrast is *high*. The contrast of an image is changed by changing the slope of the graph[1]:

$$g(x, y) = a \cdot f(x, y) \tag{4.2}$$

If $a > 1$ the contrast is increased and if $a < 1$ the contrast is decreased. For example, when $a = 2$ the pixels 112 and 114 will get the values 224 and 228, respectively. The difference between them is increased by a factor 2 and the contrast is therefore increased. In Fig. 4.4 the effect of changing the contrast can be seen.

If we combine the equations for brightness, Eq. 4.1, and contrast, Eq. 4.2, we have

$$g(x, y) = a \cdot f(x, y) + b, \tag{4.3}$$

which is the equation of a straight line. Let us look at an example of how to apply this equation. Say we are interested in a certain part of the input image where the

---

[1] In practice the line is not rotated around (0, 0) but rather around the center point (127, 127), hence $b = 127(1 - a)$. However, for the discussion here it suffices to say that $b = 0$ and only look at the slope.

a < 1   a = 1   a > 1

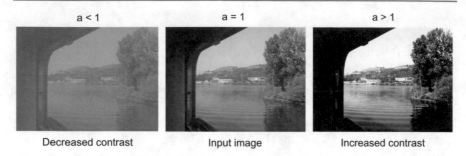

Decreased contrast   Input image   Increased contrast

Fig. 4.4 If a in Eq. 4.2 is one, the resulting image will be equal to the input image. If a is smaller than one then the resulting image will have decreased contrast, and if a is higher than one, then the resulting image will have increased contrast

contrast might not be sufficient. We therefore find the range of the pixels in this part of the image and map them to the entire range, [0, 255] in the output image. Say that the minimum pixel value and maximum pixel values in the input image are 100 and 150, respectively. Changing the contrast then means to say that all pixel value below 100 are set to zero in the output and all pixel values above 150 are set to 255 in the output image. The pixels in the range [100, 150] are then mapped to [0, 255] using Eq. 4.3 where a and b are defined as follows:

$$a = \frac{255}{f_2 - f_1} \qquad b = -a \cdot f_1, \qquad (4.4)$$

where $f_1 = 100$ and $f_2 = 150$.

Generally, a linear mapping can be used to obtain a desired minimum $v_{min,d}$ and maximum $v_{max,d}$ (without clipping). Initially, the current minimum v_{min} and v_{max} are found by going through all the pixel values in the input image. These are used to apply the mapping:

$$g(x, y) = \frac{v_{max,d} - v_{min,d}}{v_{max} - v_{min}}(f(x, y) - v_{min}) + v_{min,d}. \qquad (4.5)$$

This mapping can, for example, be used to map an arbitrary range to the interval [0; 1] and back again after performing another mapping. For example, converting a gray-scale image where the values are in the interval [0, 255] to an image where the values lie in the interval [0, 1] can be done using Eq. 4.5. Here $v_{min,d} = 0$, $v_{max,d} = 1$, $v_{min} = 0$, $v_{max} = 255$. This leads to

$$g(x, y) = \frac{1}{255} \cdot f(x, y). \qquad (4.6)$$

A pixel with value $f(x, y) = 200$ will after the mapping have value $g(x, y) = 0.784$. The inverse conversion is done using

$$g(x, y) = 255 \cdot f(x, y). \qquad (4.7)$$

We can also use a linear mapping to obtain a desired mean μ_d and standard deviation σ_d for pixel values in the image. First, the current mean μ and standard deviation σ are computed and then we apply the mapping:

$$g(x, y) = \frac{\sigma_d}{\sigma}(f(x, y) - \mu) + \mu_d. \tag{4.8}$$

Gray-level mapping is not limited to linear mappings as defined by Eq. 4.3. In fact the designer is free to define the gray-level mapping as she pleases as long as there is one and only one output value for each input value. Often the designer will utilize a well-defined graph as opposed to defining a new one, e.g., if the darker parts of the image should be enhanced a logarithmic mapping will be applied and if the bright part of the image should be enhanced an exponential mapping will be applied. This will be explored further in Sect. 4.3, but first we will take a closer look at the image histogram.

4.2 The Image Histogram

So now we know how to correct images using gray-level mapping, but how can we tell if an image is too dark or too bright?

The obvious answer is that we can simply look at the image. But we would like a more objective way of answering this question. Moreover, we are also interested in a method enabling a computer to automatically assess whether an image is too dark, too bright, or has too low a contrast, and automatically correct the image using gray-level mapping. To this end we introduce a simple but powerful tool *the image histogram*. Everybody processing images should always look at the histogram of an image before processing it—and so should you!

A histogram is a graphical representation of the frequency of events. Say you are at a party together with 85 other guests. You could then ask the age of each person and plot the result in a histogram, as illustrated in Fig. 4.5. The horizontal axis represents the possible ages and the vertical axis represents the number of people having a certain age. Each column is denoted a *bin* and the height of a bin corresponds to the number of guests having this particular age. This plot is the histogram of the age distribution among the guests at the party. If you divide each bin with the total number of samples (number of guests), each bin now represents the fraction of guests having a certain age—multiply by 100% and you have the numbers in percentages. We can, for example, see that 11.6% of the guests are 25 years old. In the rest of this book, we will denote the vertical axis in a histogram by *frequency*, i.e., the number of samples.

We now do exactly the same for the pixel values of an image. That is, we go through the entire image pixel-by-pixel and count how many pixels have the value 0, how many have the value 1, and so on up to 255. This results in a histogram with 256 bins and this is the image histogram.

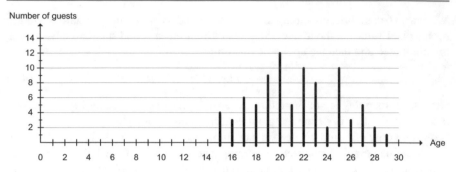

Fig. 4.5 A histogram showing the age distribution of the guests at a party. The horizontal axis represents age and the vertical axis represents the number of guests

If the majority of the pixels in an image have low values we will see this as most high bins being to the left in the histogram and can thus conclude that the image is dark. If most high bins are to the right in the histogram, the image will be bright. If the bins are spread out equally, the image will have a good contrast and vice versa. See Fig. 4.6.

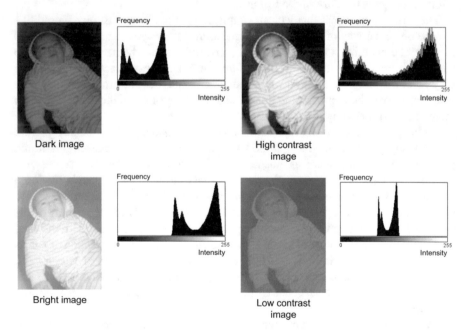

Fig. 4.6 Four images and their respective histograms. The two images to the left illustrate a too dark and a too bright image, respectively. Notice how this is reflected in the two histograms by having most bins in the low intensities and high intensities, respectively. The two images to the right illustrate good contrast and poor contrast, respectively. Again, it is important to notice that the level of contrast is also reflected in the two histograms

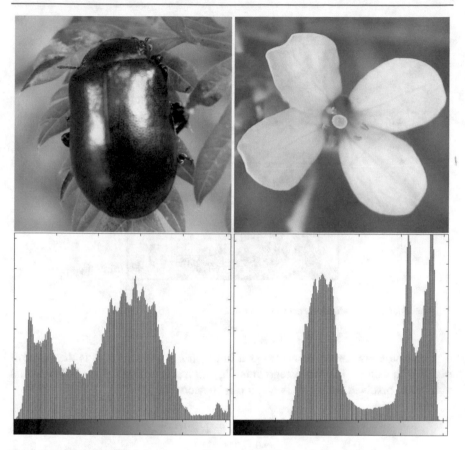

Fig. 4.7 Two images with their respective histograms. While the black beetle causes a peak in the histogram at the low values, the flower causes peaks in the high values of its histogram. In both images, the background creates a large peak in the middle of the histogram

A simple inspection of the histogram can also give some clues to the difficulties in identifying important structures in images. Two images and their histograms can be seen in Fig. 4.7. While the background in both images creates a large peak in the middle of the histogram, the peaks belonging to both the flower and the beetle can easily be identified. Later we will describe how this information is useful when converting the images into binary images using thresholding.

Note that when calculating an image histogram the actual position of the pixels is not used. This means (i) that many images have the same histogram and (ii) that an image cannot be reconstructed from the histogram. In Fig. 4.8 four images with the same histogram are shown.

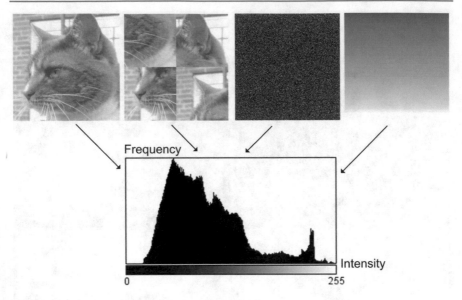

Fig. 4.8 Four images with the exact same histogram

The histogram can be described as a function $h(v)$, where $h(v)$ is the count of pixels with value v. For the histogram in Fig. 4.9 it is seen that $h(2) = 7$. If the total number of pixels in the image is N_p, it can be seen that

$$\sum_{v=0}^{255} h(v) = N_p. \tag{4.9}$$

The histogram can be *normalized* by dividing each bin count with the total number of pixels:.

$$H(v) = \frac{h(v)}{N_p}. \tag{4.10}$$

$H(v)$ is equal to a probability density function and can be seen as the probability of a pixel having value v. If a random pixel is selected from the image in Fig. 4.9, the probability of this pixel having value $v = 4$ is $\frac{6}{36} \cdot 100\% = 17\%$. As is the case with probability density functions:

$$\sum_{v=0}^{255} H(v) = 1. \tag{4.11}$$

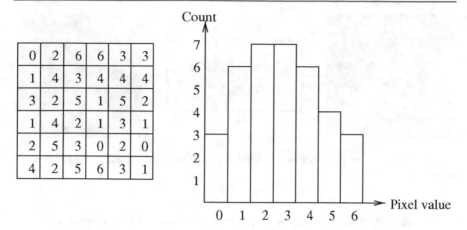

Fig. 4.9 6×6 image and its histogram. This is an example image since the gray value range is only 0–6

4.2.1 Histogram Stretching

Armed with this new tool we now seek a method to automatically correct the image so that it is neither too bright nor too dark and does not have too low contrast. In terms of histograms, this means that the histogram should start at 0 and end at 255. We obtain this by mapping the left-most non-zero bin in the histogram to 0 and the right-most non-zero bin to 255, see Fig. 4.10.

We can see that the histogram has been stretched so that the very dark and very bright values are now used. It should also be noted that the distance between the different bins is increased; hence, the contrast is improved. This operation is denoted *histogram stretching* and the algorithm is exactly the same as Eq. 4.3 with a and b defined as in Eq. 4.4. f_1 is the left-most non-zero bin in the histogram and f_2 is the right-most non-zero bin in the histogram of the input image.

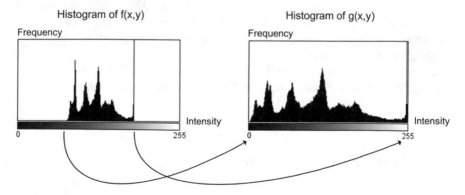

Fig. 4.10 The concept of histogram stretching

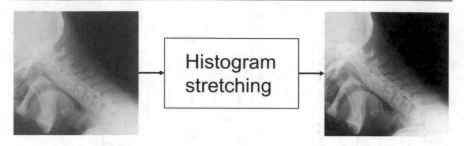

Fig. 4.11 An example of histogram stretching. It can be seen that the output image has better contrast than the input image

Conceptually it might be easier to appreciate the equation if we rearrange Eq. 4.3:

$$g(x, y) = \frac{255}{f_2 - f_1} \cdot f(x, y) - f_1 \cdot a \Leftrightarrow \qquad (4.12)$$

$$g(x, y) = \frac{255}{f_2 - f_1} \cdot (f(x, y) - f_1) \qquad (4.13)$$

First the histogram is shifted left so that f_1 is located at 0. Then each value is multiplied by a factor a so that the maximum value $f_2 - f_1$ becomes equal to 255. In Fig. 4.11 an example of histogram stretching is illustrated.

For the X-ray image shown in Fig. 4.12 to the left, $v_{min} = 32$ and $v_{max} = 208$. The linear histogram stretching can then be applied by using this equation on all pixels in the input image:

$$g(x, y) = \frac{255}{176}(f(x, y) - 32). \qquad (4.14)$$

The result can be seen in Fig. 4.12 to the right. It can be seen that histogram stretching increases the contrast in the image and makes it easier to recognize the smaller details in the finger bones. It is important to remember that histogram stretching does not change the number of occupied bins in the image histogram.

An obvious problem with histogram stretching is that it is very vulnerable to pixel value outliers. If just one pixel has the value 0 and another 255, histogram stretching will not work, since $f_2 - f_1 = 255$. A more robust method is therefore to apply *histogram equalization*. Histogram equalization is based on non-linear gray-level mapping using a *cumulative histogram*.

Imagine we have a histogram $H[i]$ where i is a bin number (between 0 and 255) and $H[i]$ is the height of bin i. The cumulative histogram is then defined as[2]:

$$C[j] = \sum_{i=0}^{j} H[i] \qquad (4.15)$$

In Table 4.1 a small example is provided.

---

[2]See Appendix B for a definition of $\sum$.

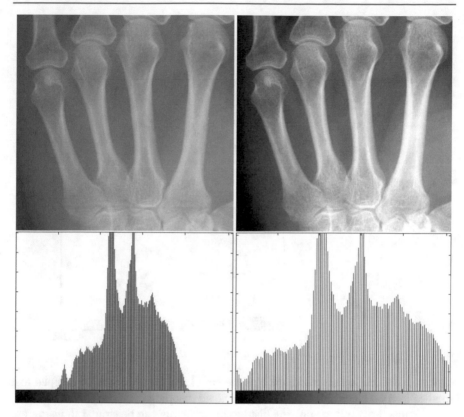

Fig. 4.12 To the left is the original X-ray image and to the right the X-ray image after histogram stretching

Table 4.1 A small histogram and its cumulative histogram. i is the bin number, $H[i]$ the height of bin i, and $C[i]$ is the height of the ith bin in the cumulative histogram

i	0	1	2	3
$H[i]$	1	5	0	7
$C[i]$	1	6	6	13

In Fig. 4.13 a histogram is shown together with its cumulative histogram. Where the histogram has high bins, the cumulative histogram has a steep slope and where the histogram has low bins, the cumulative histogram has a small slope. The idea is now to use the cumulative histogram as a gray-level mapping. So the pixel values located in areas of the histogram where the bins are high and dense will be mapping to a wider interval in the output since the slope is above 1. On the other hand, the

Fig. 4.13 An example of a cumulative histogram. Notice how the tall bins in the ordinary histogram translate into steep slopes in the cumulative histogram

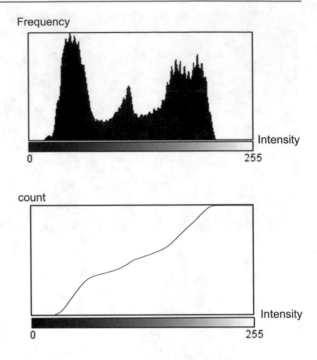

regions in the histogram where the bins are small and far apart will be mapped to a smaller interval since the slope of the gray-level mapping is below 1.

Note that the result of applying histogram stretching can be similar to histogram equalization if all insignificant bins are ignored.

4.3   Non-Linear Gray-Level Mapping

In some cases, it is not possible to achieve a good result using a linear mapping of gray values and it is necessary to use a *non-linear mapping*. In this section some of the commonly used mapping functions are described.

4.3.1   Gamma Mapping

In many cameras and display devices (flat panel televisions, for example), it is useful to be able to increase or decrease the contrast in the dark gray levels and the light gray levels individually. A commonly used non-linear mapping is gamma mapping, that is, defined for positive γ as

$$g(x, y) = f(x, y)^{\gamma}. \tag{4.16}$$

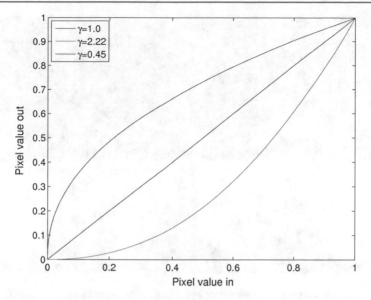

Fig. 4.14 Gamma mapping curves for different gammas

Some gamma mapping curves are illustrated in Fig. 4.14. For $\gamma = 1$ we get the identity mapping. For $0 < \gamma < 1$ we increase the dynamics in the dark areas by increasing the mid-levels. For $\gamma > 1$ we increase the dynamics in the bright areas by decreasing the mid-levels. The gamma mapping is defined so that the input and output pixel values are in the range [0, 1]. It is therefore necessary to transform the input pixel values using Eq. 4.5 before the gamma transformation. The output values should also be scaled from [0, 1] to [0, 255] after the gamma transformation.

As an example, the gray values of an X-ray image has been gamma mapped with two different gamma values. The result can be seen together with the original image in Fig. 4.15. The histograms show that a gamma value lower than one *pushes* the gray values to the right and that gamma values higher than one pushes the gray values to the left.

As another example, a pixel in a gray-scale image with value 120 is gamma mapped with $\gamma = 2.22$. Initially, the pixel value is transformed into the interval [0, 1] by dividing with 255, $v_1 = 120/255 = 0.4706$. Secondly, the gamma mapping is performed $v_2 = 0.4706^{2.22} = 0.1876$. Finally, it is mapped back to the interval [0, 255] giving the result $0.1876 \cdot 255 = 47$.

4.3.2   Logarithmic and Exponential Mapping

An alternative non-linear mapping is based on the natural logarithm operator in the following just written as log. Each pixel is replaced by the logarithm of the pixel value. This has the effect that low intensity pixel values are enhanced. It is often

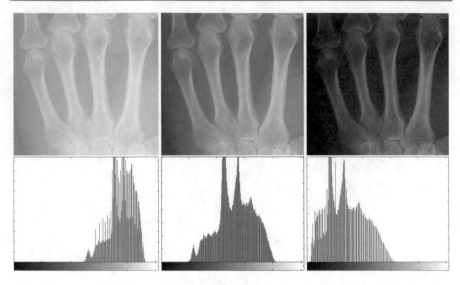

Fig. 4.15 Gamma mapping to the left with $\gamma = 0.45$ and to the right with $\gamma = 2.22$. In the middle the original image

used in cases where the dynamic range of the image is to great to be displayed or in images where there are a few very bright spots on a darker background. Since the logarithm is not defined for 0, the mapping is defined as

$$g(x, y) = c \log(1 + f(x, y)), \tag{4.17}$$

where c is a scaling constant that ensures that the maximum output value is 255 (for byte images). It is calculated as

$$c = \frac{255}{\log(1 + v_{\max})}, \tag{4.18}$$

where $v_{\max}$ is the maximum pixel value in the input image.

The behavior of the logarithmic mapping can be controlled by changing the pixel values of the input image using a linear mapping before the logarithmic mapping. The logarithmic mapping from the interval [0, 255] to [0, 255] is shown in Fig. 4.16. This mapping will clearly stretch the low intensity pixels while suppressing the contrast in high intensity pixels.

The exponential mapping uses a part of the exponential curve. It can be parameterized as

$$g(x, y) = \frac{(1 + k)^{f(x, y)} - 1}{k}, \tag{4.19}$$

where k is a parameter that can be used to change of shape of the transformation curve. The exponential mapping enhances detail in the light areas while decreasing detail in the dark areas.

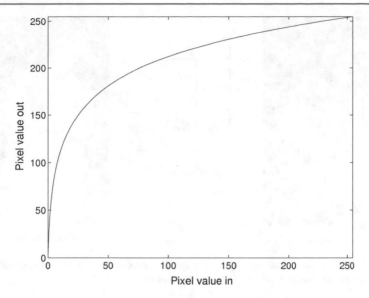

Fig. 4.16 Logarithmic mapping from the interval [0, 255] to [0, 255]

4.4 Thresholding

One of the most fundamental point processing operations is *thresholding*. Threshold-ing is the special case when $f_1 = f_2$ in Eq. 4.13. Mathematically this is undefined, but in practice it simply means that all input values below f_1 are mapped to zero in the output and all input values above f_1 are mapped to 255 in the output. This means that we will only have completely black or completely white pixel values in the output image. Such an image is denoted a *binary image*, see Fig. 4.17, and this representation of an object is denoted the *silhouette* of the object.

One might argue that we lose information when doing this operation. However, imagine you are designing a system where the goal is to find the position of a person in a sequence of images and use that to control some parameter in a game. In such a situation all you are interested in is the position of the human and nothing more. In this case, thresholding in such a manner that the person is white and the rest is black would be exactly what we are interested in. In fact, we can say we have removed the redundant information or eliminated noise in the image.

Thresholding is normally not described in terms of gray-level mapping, but rather as the following *segmentation* algorithm:

$$\begin{array}{l} \text{if } f(x, y) \leq T \text{ then g(x,y)} = 0 \\ \text{if } f(x, y) > T \text{ then g(x,y)} = 255 \end{array} \text{'} \qquad (4.20)$$

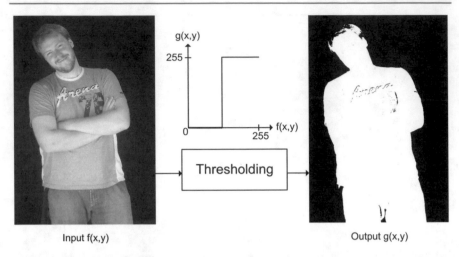

Input f(x,y)   Output g(x,y)

Fig. 4.17 An example of thresholding. Notice that it is impossible to define a perfect silhouette with the thresholding algorithm. This is in general the case

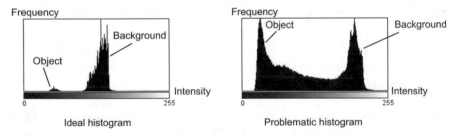

Ideal histogram   Problematic histogram

Fig. 4.18 Ideal histogram (bimodal): a clear definition of object and background. Problematic histogram: the distinction between the object and the background is harder, if not impossible. Note that objects are dark on a light background in this example

where T is the threshold value. We might of course also reverse the equalities so that every pixel below the threshold value is mapped to white and every pixel above the threshold value is mapped to black.

In many image processing systems, thresholding is a key step to segmenting the foreground (information) from the background (noise). To obtain a good thresholding the image should have a histogram which is bimodal. This means that the histogram should consist of two "mountains" where one mountain corresponds to the background pixels and the other mountain to the foreground pixels. Such a histogram is illustrated to the left in Fig. 4.18. In an ideal situation like the one shown to the right, deciding the threshold value is not critical, but in real life the two mountains are not always separated so nicely and care must therefore be taken when defining the correct threshold value.

In situations where you have influence on the image acquisition process, keep this histogram in mind. In fact, one of the sole purposes of image acquisition is often to

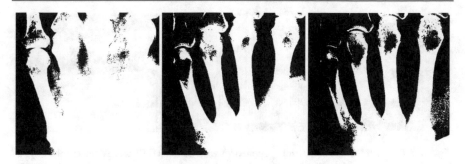

Fig. 4.19 A thresholded X-ray image of a hand. The thresholds (left to right) are 110, 128, and 140

achieve such a histogram. So it is often beneficial to develop your image processing algorithms and your setup (camera, optics, lighting, and environment) in parallel.

To evaluate if it is possible to extract the metacarpal bones from the background in an X-ray image some experimentation with thresholds is performed. In Fig. 4.12 to the left, an X-ray is seen together with the image histogram. Several peaks are noticed; however, when thresholds of 110, 128, and 140 are tried, it can be realized that it is not possible to find one threshold that can separate all bones from the background as shown in Fig. 4.19.

4.4.1 Automatic Thresholding

There exist several methods to automatically determine one or more thresholds in an image. A common method, called Otsu's method, assumes that the image contains two classes (foreground and background) and then calculates a threshold that separates these classes based on the histogram [7]. The threshold is chosen so the combined class variances are minimized. Assume that a threshold T is given, then the variance of all the pixels classified as background can be calculated together with the variance of all the object pixels. These two variance measures are combined using a set of weights (based on the number of pixels in each class) into a combined variance. It can be shown that the optimal T can be calculated very fast based on a pre-computed histogram [7].

Otsu's automatic thresholding has been applied to an abdominal CT slice as shown in Fig. 4.20. The light gray material is fat tissue and the darker gray is organ tissue (part of the liver). The methods successfully separate the two types of tissue. In this case, there are two clearly visible peaks in the histogram with a good separation, which makes the problem easy to solve. Often there is significant overlap between the pixel values of the foreground and the background.

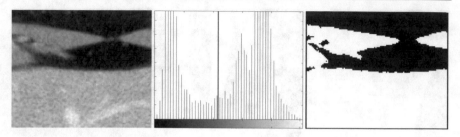

Fig. 4.20 Otsu's automatic thresholding applied on an abdominal CT slice. To the left the original CT slice, where the light gray material is fat tissue and the darker gray is organ tissue (part of the liver). In the middle the histogram and to the right the thresholded image, where the threshold was found to be 108

4.5 Image Arithmetic

Instead of combining an image with a scalar as in Eq. 4.1, an image can also be combined with another image. Say we have two images of equal size, $f_1(x, y)$ and $f_2(x, y)$. These are combined pixelwise in the following way:

$$g(x, y) = f_1(x, y) + f_2(x, y) \qquad (4.21)$$

Other arithmetic operations can also be used to combine two images, but most often addition or subtraction are the ones applied.

When adding two images some of the pixel values in the output image might have values above 255. For example, if $f_1(10, 10) = 150$ and $f_2(10, 10) = 200$, then $g(10, 10) = 350$. In principle, this doesn't matter, but if an 8-bit image is used for the output image, then we have the problem known as *overflow*. That is, the value cannot be represented. A similar situation can occur for image subtraction where a negative number can appear in the output image. This is known as *underflow*.

The solution is therefore to use a temporary image (16-bit or 32-bit) to store the result and then map the temporary image to a standard 8-bit image for further processing. This principle is illustrated in Fig. 4.21.

This algorithm is the same as used for histogram stretching except that the minimum value can be negative:

1. Find the minimum number in the temporary image, f_1
2. Find the maximum number in the temporary image, f_2
3. Shift all pixels so that the minimum value is 0: $g_i(x, y) = g_i(x, y) - f_1$
4. Scale all pixels so that the maximum value is 255: $g(x, y) = g_i(x, y) \cdot \frac{255}{f_2 - f_1}$

where $g_i(x, y)$ is the temporary image.

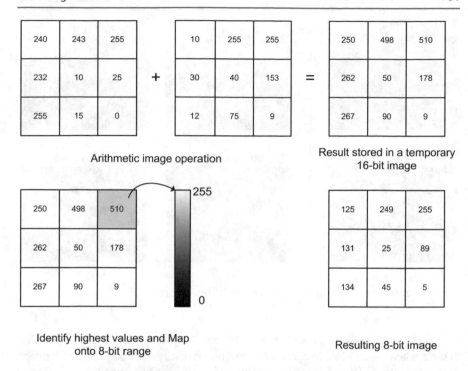

Fig. 4.21 An example of overflow and how to handle it. The addition of the images produces values above the range of the 8-bit image, which is handled by storing the result in a temporary image. In this temporary image, the highest value is identified and used to scale the intensity values down into the 8-bit range. The same approach is used for underflow. This approach also works for images with both over- and underflow

4.5.1   Applying Image Arithmetic

Image arithmetic has a number of interesting usages and here two are presented. The first one is based on image subtraction and can be used to assess your image acquisition setup. Imagine you have constructed a setup with a camera and some lighting etc. You connect a monitor and look at the images being captured by the camera. They might seem fine, but in many cases you cannot visually judge the level of noise in the setup. For example, if the camera is mounted on a table which moves slightly whenever someone is walking nearby. Another typical noise source is the fact that most lighting is powered by a $50Hz$ supply, meaning that the level of illumination changes rapidly over time. Such noise sources can often not be detected by simply looking at the scene. Instead, you subtract two consecutive images and display the result. If the images are the same, meaning no noise in the scene, then the output image (after image subtraction) should only contain zeros, hence be black. The more non-zero pixels you have in the output image the more noise is present in your setup. This method can also be combined with a histogram to provide quantitative results.

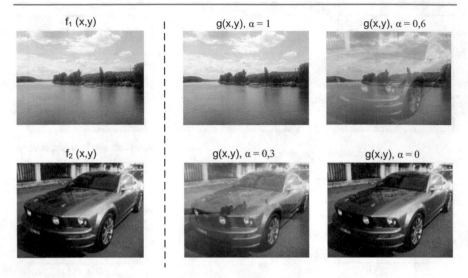

Fig. 4.22 Examples of alpha blending, with different alpha values

Another very relevant use of image arithmetic is *alpha blending*. Alpha blending is used when mixing two images, for example, gradually changing from one image to another image. The idea is to extend Eq. 4.21 so that the two images have different importance. For example, 20% of $f_1(x, y)$ and 80% of $f_2(x, y)$. Note that the sum of the two percentages should be 100%. Concretely, the equation is rewritten as

$$g(x, y) = \alpha \cdot f_1(x, y) + (1 - \alpha) \cdot f_2(x, y), \qquad (4.22)$$

where $\alpha \in [0, 1]$ and α is the Greek letter "alpha", hence the name alpha blending. If $\alpha = 0.5$ then the two images are mixed equally and Eq. 4.22 has the same effect as Eq. 4.21. In Fig. 4.22, a mixing of two images is shown for different values of α.

In Eq. 4.22, α is the same for every pixel, but it can actually be different from pixel to pixel. This means that we have an entire image (with the same size as $f_1(x, y)$, $f_2(x, y)$ and $g(x, y)$) where we have α-values instead of pixels: $\alpha(x, y)$. Such an "α-image" is often referred to as an *alpha-channel*.

4.5.2   Noise Reduction Using Pixelwise Summing

Assume that we have acquired a set of n images of a static scene and that each acquired pixel $g(x, y)$ is the sum of the true pixel value $f(x, y)$ and white Gaussian noise, i.e.,

$$g(x, y) = f(x, y) + \epsilon(x, y), \qquad (4.23)$$

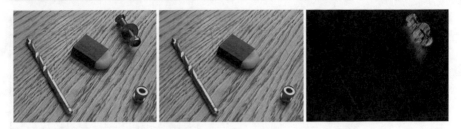

Fig. 4.23 Two images of the same scene with a small difference and the pixelwise absolute difference. In the absolute difference image, the bolt with shadow overlayed with the woodgrain texture of the table is seen

where $\epsilon(x, y) \in N(0, \sigma^2)$. After adding the n images and dividing by n we get

$$\frac{1}{n} \sum_n g(x, y) = f(x, y) + \frac{1}{n} \sum_n \epsilon(x, y), \tag{4.24}$$

where

$$\frac{1}{n} \sum_n \epsilon(i, j) \in N\left(0, \frac{\sigma^2}{n}\right). \tag{4.25}$$

We see that the noise variance has been reduced with a factor of n.

4.5.3   Motion Detection Using Pixelwise Differencing

Pixelwise absolute difference is useful for motion detection when only the object of interest moves. Assume that we have acquired two images $f_1(x, y)$ and $f_2(x, y)$ of the same scene at two different times. Then the image $|f_1(i, j) - f_2(i, j)|$ will have high values where changes have occurred and low values where nothing has happened. This is illustrated in Fig. 4.23.

4.6   Programming Point Processing Operations

When implementing one of the point processing operations in software the following is done.

Remember that each pixel is individually processed meaning that it does not matter in which order the pixels are processed. However, we follow the order illustrated in Fig. 4.24. Starting in the upper left corner we move from left to right and from top to bottom ending in the lower right corner.[3]

---

[3] Note that the above order of scanning through the image and the code example is general and used for virtually all methods, operations, and algorithms presented in this book.

Fig. 4.24 The order in
which the pixels are visited.
Illustrated for a 10×10
image

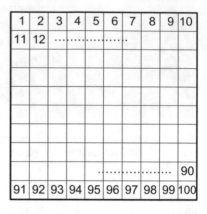

Note that this order corresponds to the way the coordinate system is defined, see Fig. 2.19. The reason for this order is that it corresponds to the order in which the pixels from the camera are sent to the memory of the computer. Also the same order the pixels on your TV are updated. Physically the pixels are also stored in this order meaning that your algorithm is faster when you process the pixels in this order due to memory access time.

In terms of programming, the point processing operations can be implemented as illustrated below—here exemplified in C-code:

Point processing code

```
for (y = 0; y < M; y = y + 1)
{
    for (x = 0; x < N; x = x + 1)
    {
        temp = GetPixel(input, x, y);
        value = Operation(temp);
        SetPixel(output, x, y, value);
    }
}
```

Here M is the height of the image and N is the width of the image. GetPixel is a function, which returns the value of the pixel at position (x, y) in the image called input. The function SetPixel changes the value of the pixel at position (x, y) in the image called output to value. Note that the two functions are not built-in C-functions. That is, you either need to write them yourself or include a library where they (or similar functions) are defined.

The programming example primarily consists of two FOR-loops which go through the image, pixel-by-pixel, in the order illustrated in Fig. 4.24. For each pixel, a point processing operation is applied.

Below we show what the C-code would look like if the operation in Eq. 4.3 were implemented.

Implementation of Eq. 4.3

```
for (y = 0; y < M; y = y + 1)
{
    for (x = 0; x < N; x = x + 1)
    {
        value = a * GetPixel(input, x, y) + b;
        SetPixel(output, x, y, value);
    }
}
```

Here a and b are defined beforehand.

Below we show what the C-code would look like if the operation in Eq. 4.20 were implemented.

Implementation of Eq. 4.20

```
for (y = 0; y < M; y = y + 1)
{
    for (x = 0; x < N; x = x + 1)
    {
        if (GetPixel(input, x, y) > T)
            SetPixel(output, x, y, 255);
        else
            SetPixel(output, x, y, 0);
    }
}
```

Here the threshold value, T, is defined beforehand.

Neighborhood Processing

5

In the previous chapter we saw that a pixel value in the output was set according to a pixel value in the input *at the same position* and a point processing operation. This principle has many useful applications (as we saw), but it cannot be applied to investigate the relationship between *neighboring pixels*. For example, if we look at the pixel values in the small area in Fig. 5.1, we can see that a significant change in intensity values occurs in the lower left corner. This could indicate the boundary of an object and by finding the boundary pixels we have found the object.

In this and the next chapter, we present a number of methods where the neighbor pixels play a role when determining the output value of a pixel. Overall these methods are denoted *neighborhood processing* and the principle is illustrated in Fig. 5.2. The value of a pixel in the output is determined by the value of the pixel at the same position in the input *and* the neighbors together with a neighborhood processing operation. We use the same notation as in the previous chapter, i.e., $f(x, y)$ is the input image and $g(x, y)$ is the output image.[1]

5.1 The Median Filter

If we look at Fig. 5.3, we can see that it has been infected with some kind of noise (the black and white dots). Let us set out to remove this noise. First of all, we zoom in on the image and look closer at particular pixel values. What we can see is that the noise is isolated pixels having a value of either 0 (black) or 255 (white), such

---

[1]Readers unfamiliar with vectors and matrices are advised to consult Appendix B before reading this chapter.

© Springer Nature Switzerland AG 2020
R. R. Paulsen and T. B. Moeslund, *Introduction to Medical Image Analysis*,
Undergraduate Topics in Computer Science,
https://doi.org/10.1007/978-3-030-39364-9_5

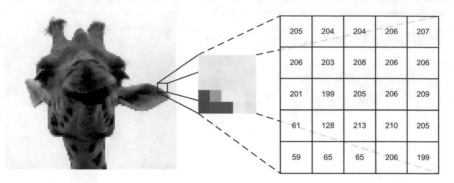

Fig. 5.1 A part of the giraffe image has been enlarged to show the edge which humans easily perceive. Using methods described in this chapter the computer will also be able to tell where the edge is

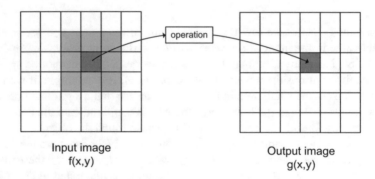

Input image
f(x,y)

Output image
g(x,y)

Fig. 5.2 The principle of neighborhood processing. To calculate a pixel in the output image, a pixel from the input image and its neighbors are processed

noise is denoted *salt-and-pepper noise*. By *isolated* we mean that they have a value very different from their neighbors. We need somehow to identify such pixels and replace them by a value which is more similar to the neighbors.

One solution is to replace the noise pixel by the *mean* value of the neighbors. Say we use the eight nearest neighbors for the noise pixel at position (1, 1) in the image patch in Fig. 5.3. To not lose the information, the actual pixel is also included. The mean value is then (using nine pixels in total):

$$\text{Mean value} = \frac{205 + 204 + 204 + 206 + 0 + 208 + 201 + 199 + 205}{9} = 181.3$$

This results in the noise pixel being replaced by 181 (since we convert the value 181.3 to the integer value 181), which is more similar to the neighbors. However, the value still stands out and therefore the *median* is often used instead. The median value of a group of numbers is found by ordering the numbers in increasing order

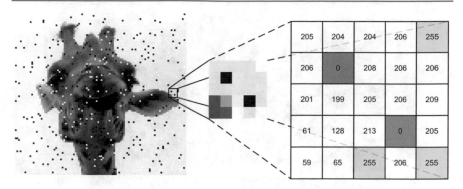

Fig. 5.3 An image infected with salt-and-pepper noise. The noise is easily recognized in both the image and the number representation

and picking the middle value. Say we use the eight nearest neighbors for the first pixel infested by noise in Fig. 5.3 (and also include the pixel itself). The ordering yields

Ordering : [0, 199, 201, 204, *204*, 205, 205, 206, 208]   Median = 204

and the middle value is 204; hence, the median is 204. The noise pixel is now replaced by 204, which does not stand out.

The next question is how to find the noise pixels in order to know where to perform the median operation. For the particular example, we could scan the image pixel-by-pixel and look for isolated values of 0 or 255. When encountered, the median operation could be applied. In general, however, a pixel with a value of say 234 could also be considered noise if it is isolated (stands out from its neighbors). Therefore, the median operation is applied to every single pixel in the image and we call this *filtering the image* using a *median filter*. Filtering the image refers to the process of applying a filter (here the median filter) to the entire image. It is important to note that by filtering the image we apply the filter to each and every pixel.

When filtering the image we of course need to decide which operation to apply but we also need to specify the size of the filter. The filter used in Fig. 5.2 is a 3×3 filter. Since filters are centered on a particular pixel (the center of the filter) the size of the filter is uneven, i.e., 3, 5, 7, etc. Very often filters have equal spatial dimensions, i.e., $3 \times 3, 5 \times 5, 7 \times 7$, etc. Sometimes a filter is described by its radius rather than its size. The radius of a 3×3 filter is 1, 2 for a 5×5 filter, 3 for a 7×7 filter, etc. The radius/size of a filter controls the number of neighbors included. The more neighbors included, the more strongly the image is filtered. Whether this is desirable or not depends on the application. Note that the larger the size, the more processing power is required by the computer. Applying a filter to an image is done by scanning through the image pixel-by-pixel from the upper left corner toward the lower right corner, as described in the previous chapter. Figure 5.4 shows how the

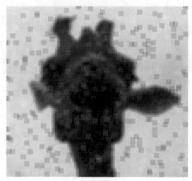 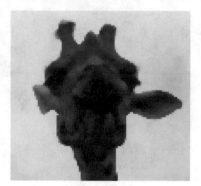

Mean filtered   Median filtered

Fig. 5.4 Resulting images of two noise filters. Notice that the mean filter does not remove all the noise and that it blurs the image. The median filter removes all the noise and only blurs the image slightly

image in Fig. 5.3 is being filtered by a 3×3 (radius = 1) mean and median filter, respectively. Note the superiority of the median filter.

In terms of programming, the Median filter can be implemented as illustrated below—here exemplified in C-code[2]:

Implementation of the median filter

```
for (y = Radius; y < (M - Radius); y = y + 1)
{
    for (x = Radius; x < (N - Radius); x = x + 1)
    {
        GetPixelValues(x, y);
        SortPixelValues();
        value = FindMedian();
        SetPixel(output, x, y, value);
    }
}
```

Here M is the height of the image, N is the width of the image and Radius is the radius of the filter. The function GetPixelValues receives an array of pixel values in the area defined by Radius around the pixel with coordinates (x,y).

What should be noticed both in the figure and in the code is that the output image will be smaller than the input image. The reason is that the filter is defined with a center and a radius, but if the center is a pixel in, for example, the first row, then no

---

[2]This implementation is just an example. The median filter can be implemented much more efficient.

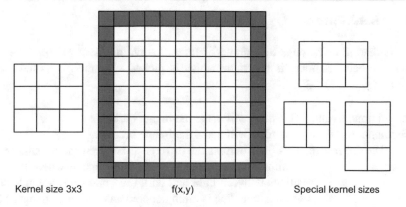

Kernel size 3x3   f(x,y)   Special kernel sizes

Fig. 5.5 An illustration of the border problem, which occurs when using neighborhood processing algorithms. If a kernel with a size of 3×3 is used, then the border illustrated in $f(x, y)$ cannot be processed. One solution to this is to apply kernels with special sizes on the borders, like the ones showed to the right

neighbors are defined above. This is known as the *border problem*, see Fig. 5.5. If it is unacceptable that the output image is reduced in size (for example, because it is to be added to the input image), then inspiration can be found in one of the following suggestions[3]:

Increase the output image	After the output image has been generated, the pixel values in the last row (if radius = 1) are duplicated and appended to the image. The same for the first row, first column, and last column.
Increase the input image	Before the image is filtered, the pixel values in the last row (if radius = 1) of the input image are duplicated and appended to the input image. The same for the first row, first column, and last column.
Apply special filters at the rim of the image	Special filters with special sizes are defined and applied accordingly, see Fig. 5.5.

---

[3]Note that this issue is common for all neighborhood processing methods.

5.1.1 Rank Filters

The Median filter belongs to a group of filters known as *Rank Filters*. The only difference between them is the value which is picked after the pixels have been sorted:

The minimum value This filter will make the image darker.

The maximum value This filter will make the image brighter.

The difference This filter outputs the difference between the maximum and minimum value and the result is an image where the transitions between light and dark (and opposite) are enhanced. Such a transition is often denoted an edge in an image. More on this in Sect. 5.2.2.

5.2 Correlation

Correlation is an operation which also works by scanning through the image and applying a filter to each pixel. In correlation, however, the filter is denoted a *kernel* and plays a more active role. First of all the kernel is filled by numbers—denoted *kernel coefficients*. These coefficients weight the pixel value they are covering and the output of the correlation is a sum of weighted pixel values. In Fig. 5.6 some different kernels are shown.

Similar to the median filter the kernel is centered above the pixel position whose value we are calculating. We denote this center $(0, 0)$ in the kernel coordinate system and the kernel as $h(x, y)$, see Fig. 5.7. To calculate the output value we take the value of $h(-1, -1)$ and multiply it by the pixel value beneath. Let's say that we are calculating the output value of the pixel at position $(2, 2)$. Then $h(-1, -1)$ will be above the pixel $f(1, 1)$ and the values of these two pixels are multiplied together. The

1	4	7	4	1
4	16	26	16	4
7	26	41	26	7
4	16	26	16	4
1	4	7	4	1

1	1	1
1	1	1
1	1	1

2	1	0
1	0	-1
0	-1	-2

3x3 Mean kernel   5x5 Gaussian kernel   3x3 Sobel kernel

Fig. 5.6 Three different kernels

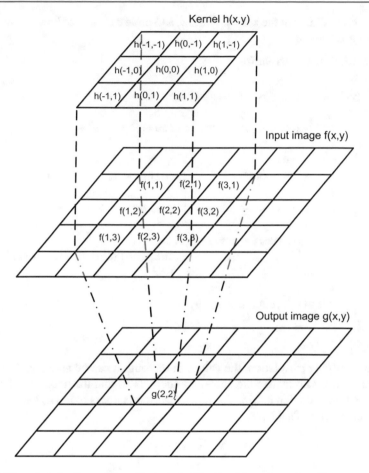

Fig. 5.7 The principle of correlation, illustrated with a 3×3 kernel on a 6×6 image

result is added to the product of the next kernel element $h(0, -1)$ and the pixel value beneath $f(2, 1)$, etc. The final value which will be written into the output image as $g(2, 2)$ is found as

$$g(2, 2) =$$
$$h(-1, -1) \cdot f(1, 1) + h(0, -1) \cdot f(2, 1) + h(1, -1) \cdot f(3, 1)+$$
$$h(-1, 0) \cdot f(1, 2) + h(0, 0) \cdot f(2, 2) + h(1, 0) \cdot f(3, 2)+$$
$$h(-1, 1) \cdot f(1, 3) + h(0, 1) \cdot f(2, 3) + h(1, 1) \cdot f(3, 3) \tag{5.1}$$

The principle is illustrated in Fig. 5.7. We say that we correlate the input image $f(x, y)$ with the kernel $h(x, y)$ and the result is $g(x, y)$. Mathematically this is expressed as $g(x, y) = f(x, y) \circ h(x, y)$ and written as

$$g(x, y) = \sum_{j=-R}^{R} \sum_{i=-R}^{R} h(i, j) \cdot f(x + i, y + j), \tag{5.2}$$

where R is the radius of the kernel.[4] Below, a C-code example of how to implement correlation is shown:

Implementation of correlation

```
for (y = Radius; y < (M - Radius); y = y + 1)
{
    for (x = Radius; x < (N - Radius); x = x + 1)
    {
        temp = 0;
        for (j = -Radius; j < (Radius + 1); j = j + 1)
        {
            for (i = -Radius; i < (Radius+1); i = i + 1)
            {
                temp = temp +
                    h(i,j) * GetPixel(input,x+i,y+j);
            }
        }
        SetPixel(output, x, y, temp);
    }
}
```

When applying correlation, the values in the output can be above 255. If this is the case, then we normalize the kernel coefficients so that the maximum output of the correlation operation is 255. The normalization factor is found as the sum of the kernel coefficients. That is,

$$\sum_x \sum_y h(x, y). \tag{5.3}$$

For the left-most kernel in Fig. 5.6 the normalization factor becomes $1 + 1 + 1 + 1 + 1 + 1 + 1 + 1 + 1 = 9$ and the resulting kernel coefficients are $1/9$ as opposed to 1.

Looking back on the previous section, we can now see that the left-most kernel in Fig. 5.6 is exactly the mean filter. The mean filter smoothes or blurs the image which has different applications. In Fig. 5.8 one application is shown where the mean filter is applied within the white box in order to hide the identity of a person. The bigger the kernel, the more the smoothing. Another type of mean filter is when a kernel like the middle one in Fig. 5.6 is applied. This provides higher weights to pixels close to the center of the kernel. This mean filter is known as a *Gaussian filter*, since the kernel coefficients are calculated from the Gaussian distribution (a bell-shaped curve).

---

[4]The reader is encouraged to play around with this equation in order to fully comprehend it.

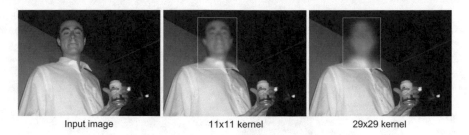

Input image   11x11 kernel   29x29 kernel

Fig. 5.8 An example of how a mean filter can be used to hide the identity of a person. The size of the mean kernel decides the strength of the filter. Actual image size: 512×384

5.2.1 Template Matching

An important application of correlation is *template matching*. Template matching is used to locate an object in an image. When applying template matching the kernel is denoted a *template*. It operates by defining an image of the object we are looking for. This object is now the template (kernel) and by correlating an image with this template, the output image indicates where the object is. Each pixel in the output image now holds a value, which states the similarity between the template and an image patch (with the same size as the template) centered at this particular pixel position. The brighter a value the higher the similarity.

In Fig. 5.9 the correlation-based template matching is illustrated. We can see a bright spot in the center of the upper part of the output corresponding to where the template matches best. Note also that as the template is shifted left and right with respect to this position, a number of bright spots appear. The distances between these spots correspond to the distance between the letters in the text.

Since correlation is based on multiplying the template and the input image, bright areas in the input image tend to produce high values in the output. This is illustrated in Fig. 5.10 where the large white section in the clothing of the child in the middle

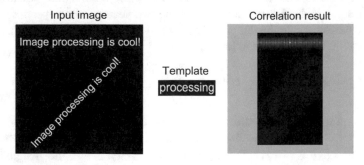

Fig. 5.9 Template matching performed by correlating the input image with a template. The result of template matching is seen to the right. The gray outer region illustrates the pixels that cannot be processed due to the border problem

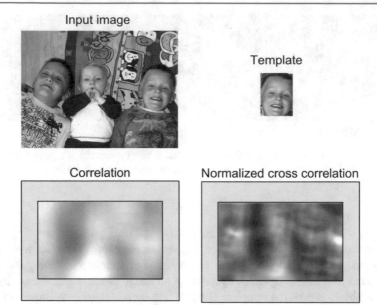

Input image

Template

Correlation

Normalized cross correlation

Fig. 5.10 Template matching using correlation and normalized cross correlation. The gray regions illustrate the pixels that cannot be processed due to the border problem

produces the highest values in the output. This problem in general makes it difficult, and in this particular case impossible, to actually find the position of the object by looking at the values in the output image.

To avoid this problem we need to normalize the values in the output so they are independent of the overall level of light in the image. To assist us in doing so we use a small trick. Let us denote the template H and the image patch F. These are both matrices, but by rearranging we can easily convert each matrix into a vector by concatenating each row (or column) in the matrix, i.e., $\vec{H}$ and $\vec{F}$.

If we now look at correlation in terms of this vector representation, we can see that Eq. 5.2 is actually the dot product between the two vectors, see Appendix B. From geometry we know that the dot product between two vectors can be normalized to the interval $[-1, 1]$ using the follow equation:

$$\cos \theta = \frac{\vec{H} \bullet \vec{F}}{|\vec{H}| \cdot |\vec{F}|}, \tag{5.4}$$

where θ is the angle between the two vectors, and $|\vec{H}|$ and $|\vec{F}|$ are the lengths of the two vectors. The normalization of the dot product between the vectors is a fact because $\cos \theta \in [-1, 1]$. The length of $|\vec{H}|$, which is also the "length" of the template, is calculated as

$$\text{Length of template} = \sqrt{\sum_{j=-R}^{R} \sum_{i=-R}^{R} h(i, j) \cdot h(i, j)}, \qquad (5.5)$$

where R is the radius of the template and $h(i, j)$ is the coefficient in the template at position (i, j). The length of the image patch is calculated in the same manner.

When using this normalization the bright spots in the output no longer depend on whether the image is bright or not but only on how similar the template and the underlying image patch are. This version of template matching is denoted *Normalized Cross Correlation* (NCC) and calculated for each pixel (x, y) using the following equation:

$$\text{NCC}(x, y) = \frac{\text{Correlation}}{\text{Length of image patch} \cdot \text{Length of template}}$$

that after inserting the relevant equations becomes

$$\text{NCC}(x, y) = \frac{\sum_{j=-R}^{R} \sum_{i=-R}^{R} (H \cdot F)}{\sqrt{\sum_{j=-R}^{R} \sum_{i=-R}^{R} (F \cdot F)} \cdot \sqrt{\sum_{j=-R}^{R} \sum_{i=-R}^{R} (H \cdot H)}}, \qquad (5.6)$$

where R is the radius of the template, $H = h(i, j)$ is the template and $F = f(x + i, y + j)$ is the image patch. $\cos \theta \in [-1, 1]$ but since the image patch and the template always contain positive numbers, $\cos \theta \in [0, 1]$, i.e., the output of normalized cross correlation is normalized to the interval $[0, 1]$, where 0 means no similarity and 1 means a complete similarity. In Fig. 5.10 the benefit of applying normalized cross correlation can be seen.

An even more advanced version of template matching exists. Here the mean values of the template and image patch are subtracted from H and F, respectively. This is known as the *zero-mean normalized cross correlation* or the *correlation coefficient*. The output is in the interval $[-1, 1]$ where 1 indicates a maximum similarity (as for NCC) and −1 indicates a maximum *negative* similarity, meaning the same pattern but opposite gray-scale values: 255 instead of 0, 254 instead of 1, etc.

Independent of the type of template matching, the kernel (template) is usually much bigger than the kernels/filters used in other neighborhood operations. Template matching is therefore a time consuming method and can benefit from introducing a region-of-interest, see Sect. 2.4.2.

A general assumption in template matching is that the object we are looking for has roughly the same size and rotation in both the template and the image. If this cannot be ensured, then we need to have multiple scaled and rotated versions of the template and perform template matching using each of these templates. This requires significant resources and the speed of the system is likely to drop.

5.2.2 Edge Detection

Another important application of correlation is *edge detection*. An edge in an image is defined as a position where a significant change in gray-level values occurs. In Fig. 5.11 an image is shown to the left. We now take an image slice defined by the vertical line between the two arrows. This new image will have the same height as the input image, but only be one pixel wide. In the figure, this is illustrated. Note that we have made it wider in order to be able to actually see it. Imagine now that we interpret the intensity values as height values. This gives us a different representation of the image, which is shown in the graph to the right.

What can be seen in the graph is that locations in the original image where we have a significant change in gray-scale value appear as significant changes in height. Such positions are illustrated by circles in the figure. It is these positions where we say we have an edge in an image.

Edges are useful in many applications since they define the contour of an object and are less sensitive to changes in the illumination compared to, for example, thresholding. Moreover, in many industrial applications image processing (or rather machine vision) is used to measure some dimensions of objects. It is therefore of great importance to have a clear definition of where an object starts and ends. Edges are often used for this purpose.

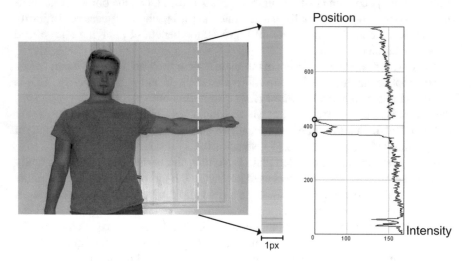

Fig. 5.11 A single column of the image is enlarged and presented in a graph. This graph contains two very significant changes in height, the position of which is marked with circles on the graph. This is how edges are defined in an image

Fig. 5.12 A curve and the tangent at four points

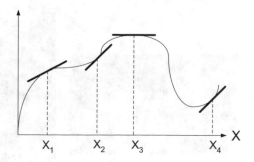

5.2.2.1 Gradients

To enable edge detection we utilize the concept of gradients. We first present gradients for a general curve and then turn to gradients in images. In the 1D case, we can define the gradient of a point as the slope of the curve at this point. Concretely this corresponds to the slope of the tangent at this point. In Fig. 5.12 the tangents of several different points are shown.

If we represent an image by height as opposed to intensity, see Fig. 5.13, then edges correspond to places where we have steep hills. For each point in this image landscape we have two gradients: one in the x-direction and one in the y-direction. Together these two gradients span a plane, known as the *tangent plane*, which intersects the point. The resulting gradient is defined as a vector

$$\nabla f(x, y) = \overrightarrow{G}(g_x, g_y), \tag{5.7}$$

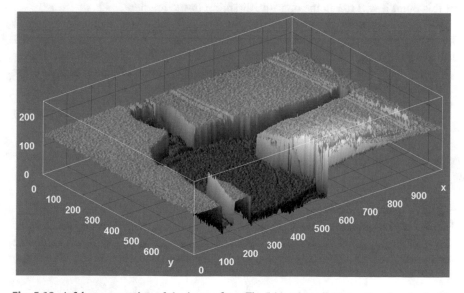

Fig. 5.13 A 3d representation of the image from Fig. 5.11, where the intensity of each pixel is interpreted as a height

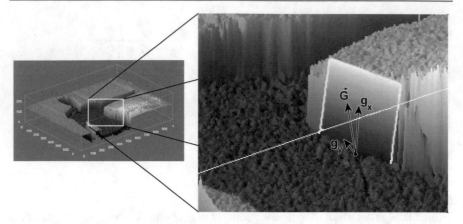

Fig. 5.14 In a 3d representation of an image, a tangent plane is present for each point. Such a plane is defined by two gradient vectors in x- and y-direction, respectively. Here the tangent plane is shown for one pixel

where g_x is the gradient in the x-direction and g_y is the gradient in the y-direction. This resulting gradient lies in the tangent plane, see Fig. 5.14. The symbol, ∇, called *nabla* is often used to describe the gradient.

We can consider $\vec{G}(g_x, g_y)$ as the direction with the steepest slope (or least steepest slope depending on how we calculate it), or in other words, if you are standing at this position in the landscape, you need to follow the opposite direction of the gradient in order to get down fastest. Or in yet another way, when water falls at this point it will run in the opposite direction of the gradient.

Besides a direction the gradient also has a *magnitude*. The magnitude expresses how steep the landscape is in the direction of the gradient, or how fast the water will run away (if you go skiing you will know that the magnitude of the gradient usually defines the difficulty of the piste). The magnitude is the length of the gradient vector and calculated as

$$\text{Magnitude} = \sqrt{g_x^2 + g_y^2} \tag{5.8}$$

$$\text{Approximated magnitude} = |g_x| + |g_y|, \tag{5.9}$$

where the approximation is introduced to achieve a faster implementation.

5.2.2.2 Image Edges

For the curves shown above, the gradients are found as the first order derivatives. This can only be calculated for continuous curves and since an image has a discrete representation (we only have pixel values at discrete positions: 0, 1, 2, 3, 4, etc.)

Prewitt

Vertical

-1	0	1
-1	0	1
-1	0	1

Horizontal

-1	-1	-1
0	0	0
1	1	1

Sobel

Vertical

-1	0	1
-2	0	2
-1	0	1

Horizontal

-1	-2	-1
0	0	0
1	2	1

Fig. 5.15 Prewitt and Sobel kernels

we need an approximation. Recalling that the gradient is the slope at a point we can define the gradient as the difference between the previous and next value. Concretely we have the following image gradient approximations:

$$g_x(x, y) \approx f(x + 1, y) - f(x - 1, y) \tag{5.10}$$

$$g_y(x, y) \approx f(x, y + 1) - f(x, y - 1) \tag{5.11}$$

We have included (x, y) in the definition of the gradients to indicate that the gradient values depend on their spatial position. This approximation will produce positive gradient values when the pixels change from dark to bright and negative values when a reversed edge is present. This will of course be opposite if the signs are switched, i.e., $g_x(x, y) \approx f(x - 1, y) - f(x + 1, y)$ and $g_y(x, y) \approx f(x, y - 1) - f(x, y + 1)$. Normally the order does not matter as we will see below.

Equation 5.10 is applied to each pixel in the input image. Concretely this is done using correlation. We correlate the image with a 1×3 kernel containing the following coefficients: $-1, 0, 1$. Calculating the gradient using this kernel is often too sensitive to noise in the image and the neighbors are therefore often also included into the kernel. The most well-known kernels for edge detection are illustrated in Fig. 5.15: the *Prewitt kernels* and the *Sobel kernels*. The difference is that the Sobel kernels weight the row and column pixels of the center pixel more than the rest.

Correlating the two Sobel kernels with the image in Fig. 5.11 yields the edge images in Fig. 5.16. The image to the left enhances horizontal edges while the image to the right enhances vertical edges. To produce the final edge image we use Eq. 5.8. That is, we first calculate the absolute value[5] of each pixel in the two images and then add them together. The result is the final edge enhanced image. After this, the final task is often to binarize the image, so that edges are white and the rest is black. This is done by a standard thresholding algorithm. In Fig. 5.16 the final edge enhanced image is shown together with binary edge images obtained using different thresholds. The choice of threshold depends on the application.

---

[5] A definition of the *absolute value* can be found in Appendix B.

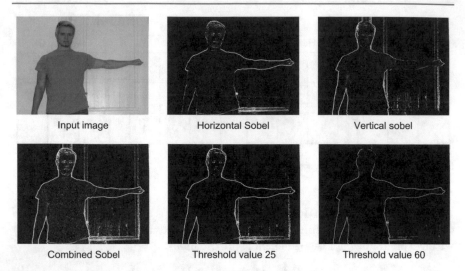

Fig. 5.16 Sobel kernels applied to an image. Each individual kernel finds edges that the other does not find. When they are combined a very nice resulting edge is created. Depending on the application, the threshold value can be manipulated to include or exclude the vaguely defined edges

5.3 Correlation Versus Convolution

The following text is likely to confuse you! One could therefore argue that it should be ignored, but we feel it is important to know the difference between correlation and *convolution* since both names are used throughout the image processing literature.

Convolution is very similar to correlation and only differs by the way the kernel is applied to the image beneath it. Mathematically convolution is defined as

$$g(x, y) = \sum_{j=-R}^{R} \sum_{i=-R}^{R} h(i, j) \cdot f(x - i, y - j) \tag{5.12}$$

Comparing this to the equation for correlation in Eq. 5.2 we can see that the only differences are the two minus signs. The interpretation of these is that the kernel is rotated 180° before doing a correlation. In Fig. 5.17 examples of rotated kernels are shown. What we can see is that symmetric kernels are equal before and after rotation, and hence convolution and correlation produce the same result. Edge detection kernels are not symmetric. However, since we often only are interested in the absolute value of an edge the correlation and convolution again yield the same result.

When applying smoothing filters, finding edges, etc. the process is often denoted convolution even though it is often implemented as correlation! When doing template matching it is virtually always denoted correlation.

1	1	1
1	1	1
1	1	1

-1	-2	-1
0	0	0
1	2	1

1	2	3
4	5	6
7	8	9

Kernels

1	1	1
1	1	1
1	1	1

1	2	1
0	0	0
-1	-2	-1

9	8	7
6	5	4
3	2	1

180° Rotated Kernels

Fig. 5.17 Three kernels and their rotated counterparts

One might rightfully ask why convolution is used in the first place. The answer is that from a general signal processing[6] point of view we actually do convolution, and correlation is convolution done with a rotated kernel. However, since correlation is easier to explain and since it is most often what is done in practice, it has been presented as though it were the other way around in this (and many other) texts. The technical reasons for the definition of convolution are beyond the scope of this text and the interested reader is referred to a general signal processing textbook.

---

[6]Image processing is a subset of signal processing.

Morphology

6

One important branch of neighborhood processing is *mathematical morphology*—or simply *morphology*. It is applicable to both gray-scale images as well as binary images, but in this text only operations related to binary images are covered. Morphology on binary images has a number of applications and in Fig. 6.1 three typical ones are illustrated. The first two illustrate how to remove the noise that very often is a side effect of thresholding. Remember that thresholding is a global operation meaning that all pixels, independent of position, are compared to the same threshold value. But if the light in the scene is not uniform or the objects have different colors (due to, for example, clothing), then we cannot define one perfect threshold value and the result is under-segmentation in some regions and over-segmentation in other regions. The left-most figure illustrates over-segmentation in the form of the small objects in the image. Under-segmentation is illustrated in the middle figure as holes inside the object. The problems associated with thresholding were also mentioned in Chap. 4 where it could be seen as the *problematic histogram* in Fig. 4.18.

The right-most example in Fig. 6.1 illustrates a problem which is related to the next chapter, where we will start to analyze individual objects. To this end we need to ensure that the objects are separated from each other.

Morphology operates like the other neighborhood processing methods by applying a kernel to each pixel in the input. In morphology, the kernel is denoted a *structuring element* and contains "0"s and "1"s. You can design the structuring element as you please, but normally the pattern of "1"s form a box or a disc. In Fig. 6.2 different sized structuring elements are visualized. Which type and size to use is up to the designer, but in general a box-shaped structuring element tends to preserve sharp object corners, whereas a disc-shaped structuring element tends to round the corners of the objects.

A structuring element is *not* applied in the same way as we saw in the previous chapter for the kernels. Instead of using multiplications and additions in the calcula-

© Springer Nature Switzerland AG 2020
R. R. Paulsen and T. B. Moeslund, *Introduction to Medical Image Analysis*,
Undergraduate Topics in Computer Science,
https://doi.org/10.1007/978-3-030-39364-9_6

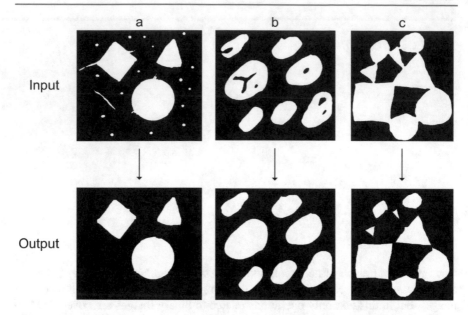

Fig. 6.1 Three examples of the uses of morphology. **a** Removing small objects. **b** Filling holes. **c** Isolating objects

tions, a structuring element is applied using either a *Hit* or a *Fit* operation. Applying one of these operations to each pixel in an image is denoted *Dilation* and *Erosion*, respectively. Combining these two methods can result in powerful image processing tools known as *Compound Operations*. We can say that there exist three levels of operation, see Fig. 6.3, and in the following, these three levels will be described one at a time. Note that for simplicity, we will in this chapter represent white as 1 instead of 255.

6.1   Level 1: Hit and Fit

The structuring element is placed on top of the image as was the case for the kernels in the previous chapter. The center of the structuring element is placed at the position of the pixel in focus and it is the value of this pixel that will be calculated by applying the structuring element. After having placed the structuring element we can apply one of two methods: Hit or Fit.

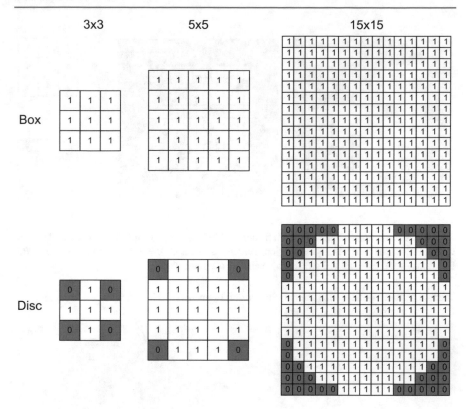

Fig. 6.2 Two types of structuring elements at different sizes

Fig. 6.3 The three levels of operation involved in morphology

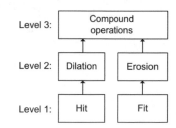

6.1.1 Hit

For each "1" in the structuring element we investigate whether the pixel at the same position in the image is also a "1". If this is the case for just one of the "1"s in the structuring element, we say that the structuring element *hits* the image at the pixel position in question (the one on which the structuring element is centered). This pixel is therefore set to "1" in the output image. Otherwise it is set to "0". In Fig. 6.4 and Table 6.1 the hit operation is illustrated with two different structuring elements.

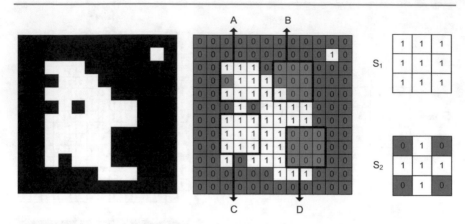

Fig. 6.4 A binary image illustrated both by colors (black and white) and numbers (0 and 1). A, B, C, and D illustrate four 3 × 3 image regions centered at: A: f(3, 3), B: f(7, 3), C: f(3, 7), and D: f(8, 8). Lastly, two different 3 × 3 structuring elements are illustrated

Table 6.1 Results of applying the two Structuring Elements (SE) in Fig. 6.4 to the input image in Fig. 6.4 at four positions: A, B, C, and D

Position	SE	Fit	Hit
A	S_1	No	Yes
A	S_2	No	Yes
B	S_1	No	Yes
B	S_2	No	No
C	S_1	Yes	Yes
C	S_2	Yes	Yes
D	S_1	No	No
D	S_2	No	No

6.1.2   Fit

For each "1" in the structuring element we investigate whether the pixel at the same position in the image is also a "1". If this is the case for *all* the "1"s in the structuring element, we say that the structuring element *fits* the image at the pixel position in question (the one on which the structuring element is centered). This pixel is therefore set to "1" in the output image. Otherwise it is set to "0". In Fig. 6.4 and Table 6.1 the fit operation is illustrated with two different structuring elements. Below we show C-code for the fit operation using a 3 × 3 box-shaped structuring element:

Implementation of the fit operation

```
Temp = 0;
for (j = y-1; j < (y+2); j = j+1)
{
    for (i = x-1; i< (x+2); i = i+1)
    {
        if (GetPixel(input, i, j) == 1)
            Temp = Temp + 1;
    }
}
if(Temp == 9)
    SetPixel(output, x, y, 1);
else
    SetPixel(output, x, y, 0);
```

Here (x, y) is the position of the pixel being processed.

6.2 Level 2: Dilation and Erosion

At the next level Hit or Fit is applied to every single pixel by scanning through the image as shown in Fig. 4.24. The size of the structuring element in these operations has the same importance as the kernel size did in the previous chapter. The bigger the structuring element, the bigger the effect in the image. As described in the previous chapter, we also have the border problem present here and solution strategies similar to those listed in Sect. 5.1 can be followed. For simplicity, we will ignore the border problem in this chapter.

6.2.1 Dilation

Applying Hit to an entire image is denoted *Dilation* and is written as

$$g(x, y) = f(x, y) \oplus SE \ . \tag{6.1}$$

The term *dilation* refers to the fact that the object in the binary image is increased in size. In general, dilating an image results in objects becoming bigger, small holes being filled, and objects being merged. How big the effect is depends on the size of the structuring element. It should be noticed that a large structuring element can be implemented by iteratively applying a smaller structuring element. This makes

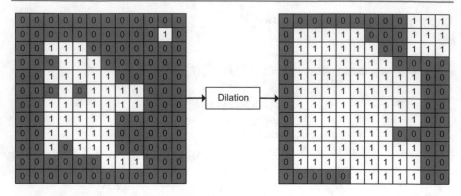

Fig. 6.5 Dilation of the binary image in Fig. 6.4 using S_1

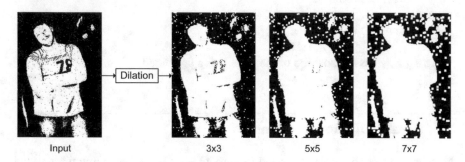

Fig. 6.6 Dilation with different sized structuring elements

sense since Eq. 6.2 holds. The equation states that dilating twice with SE_1 is similar to dilating one time with SE_2, where SE_2 is the same type but has twice the radius of SE_1. For example, if SE_2 is a 5×5 structuring element, then SE_1 is a 3×3, etc.

$$f(x, y) \oplus SE_2 \approx (f(x, y) \oplus SE_1) \oplus SE_1 . \tag{6.2}$$

In Fig. 6.5 the binary image in Fig. 6.4 is dilated using the structuring element S_1. First of all we can see that the object gets bigger. Secondly, we can observe that the hole and the convex parts of the object are filled, which makes the object more compact.

In Fig. 6.6 a real image is dilated with different sized box-shaped structuring elements. Again we can see that the object is becoming bigger and that holes inside the person are filled. What is however also apparent is that the noisy small objects are also enlarged. Below we will return to this problem.

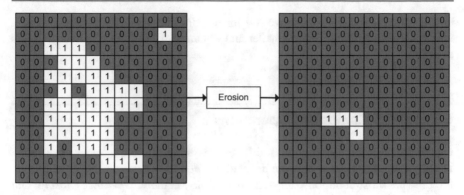

Fig. 6.7 Erosion of the binary image in Fig. 6.4 using S_1

6.2.2 Erosion

Applying Fit to an entire image is denoted Erosion and is written as

$$g(x, y) = f(x, y) \ominus SE \ . \tag{6.3}$$

The term *erosion* refers to the fact that the object in the binary image is decreased in size. In general, erosion of an image results in objects becoming smaller, small objects disappearing, and larger objects splitting into smaller objects. As for dilation the effect depends on the size of the structuring element and large structuring elements can be implemented using an equation similar to Eq. 6.2.

In Fig. 6.7 the binary image in Fig. 6.4 is eroded using the structuring element S_1. First of all, we can see that the main object gets smaller and the small objects disappear. Secondly, we can observe that the fractured parts of the main object are removed and only the "core" of the object remains. The size of this core obviously depends on the size (and shape) of the structuring element.

In Fig. 6.8 a real image is eroded with different sized box-shaped structuring elements. Again we can see that the object becomes smaller and the small (noisy)

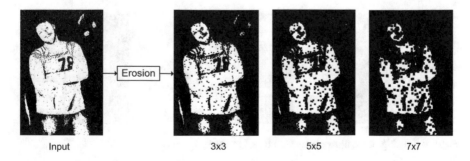

Fig. 6.8 Erosion with different sized structuring elements

objects disappear. So the price we pay for deleting the small noisy objects is that the object of interest becomes smaller and fractured. Below we will return to this problem.

6.3 Level 3: Compound Operations

Combining dilation and erosion in different ways results in a number of different image processing tools. These are denoted *compound operations*. Here we present three of the most common compound operations, namely, *Opening*, *Closing*, and *Boundary Detection*.

6.3.1 Closing

Closing deals with the problem associated with dilation, namely, that the objects increase in size when we use dilation to fill the holes in objects. This is a problem in situations where, for example, the size of the object (number of pixels) matters. The solution to this problem is luckily straight forward: we simply shrink the object by following the Dilation by an Erosion. This operation is denoted *Closing* and is written as

$$g(x, y) = f(x, y) \bullet SE = (f(x, y) \oplus SE) \ominus SE \ , \qquad (6.4)$$

where SE is the structuring element. It is essential that the structuring elements applied are exactly the same in terms of size and shape. The closing operation is said to be *idempotent*, meaning that it can only be applied one time (with the same structuring element). If applied again it has no effect whatsoever except for of course a reduced size of $g(x, y)$ due to the border problem. In Fig. 6.9, closing is illustrated for the binary image in Fig. 6.4. Closing is done with structuring element S_1. We can see that the holes and convex structures are filled; hence, the object is more compact. Moreover, the object preserves its original size.

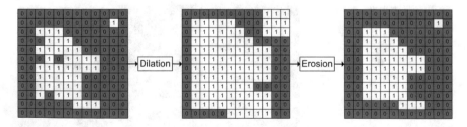

Fig. 6.9 Closing of the binary image in Fig. 6.4 using S_1

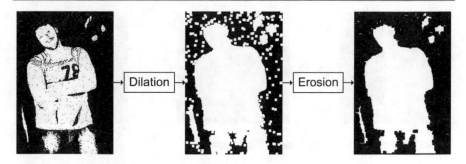

Fig. 6.10 Closing performed using 7×7 box-shaped structuring elements

In Fig. 6.10 the closing operation is applied to a real image. We can see that most internal holes are filled while the human object preserves its original size. The noisy objects in the background have not been deleted. This can be done either by the operation described just below or by finding and deleting small objects, which will be described in the next chapter.

6.3.2 Opening

Opening deals with the problem associated with erosion, namely, that the objects decrease when we use erosion to erase small noisy objects or fractured parts of bigger objects. The decreasing object size is a problem in situations where, for example, the size of the object (number of pixels) matters. The solution to this problem is luckily straight forward; we simply enlarge the object by following the erosion by dilation. This operation is denoted *Opening* and is written as

$$g(x, y) = f(x, y) \circ SE = (f(x, y) \ominus SE) \oplus SE , \tag{6.5}$$

where SE is the same structuring element. This operation is also idempotent as is the case for the closing operation. In Fig. 6.11 opening is illustrated for the binary image in Fig. 6.4. Opening is done with structuring element S_1. We can see that only a compact version of the object remains.

In Fig. 6.12 opening is applied to a real image using a 7×7 box-shaped structuring element. We can see that most noisy objects are removed while the object preserves its original size.

6.3.3 Combining Opening and Closing

In some situations we need to apply both opening and closing to an image. For example, in cases where we both have holes inside the main object *and* small noisy objects. An example is provided in Fig. 6.13. Note that the structuring elements used in the opening and the closing operations need not be the same. In Fig. 6.13

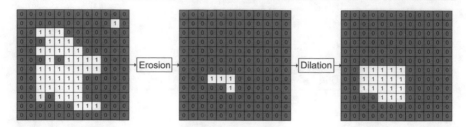

Fig. 6.11 Opening of the binary image in Fig. 6.4 using S_1

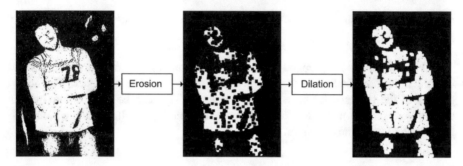

Fig. 6.12 Opening performed using a 7×7 box-shaped structuring element

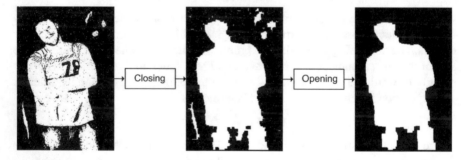

Fig. 6.13 Filtering a binary image where both holes and small noisy objects are present

the closing was performed using a 7×7 box-shaped structuring element while the opening was performed using a 15×15 box-shaped structuring element.

6.3.4   Boundary Detection

Doing edge detection in binary images is normally referred to as *boundary detection* and can be performed as described in the previous chapter. Morphology offers an alternative approach for binary images. The idea is to use erosion to make a smaller

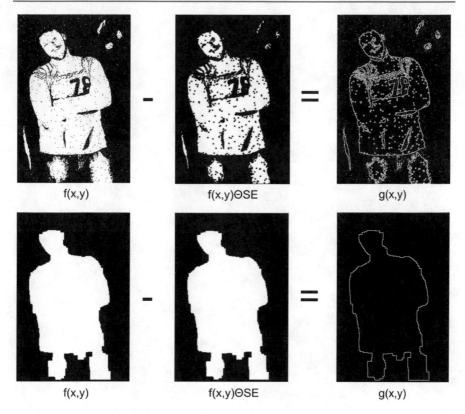

Fig. 6.14 Boundary detection

version of the object. By subtracting this from the input image only the difference stands out, namely, the boundary:

$$g(x, y) = f(x, y) - (f(x, y) \ominus SE) .\qquad(6.6)$$

If the task is only to locate the outer boundary, then the internal holes should first be filled using dilation or closing. In Fig. 6.14 examples of boundary detection are shown.

BLOB Analysis

7

Before describing what is meant by the somewhat strange title of this chapter, let us look at a few examples. In the first example the task is to design an algorithm which can figure out how many circles are present in Fig. 7.1 to the left. Obviously, the answer is three, but how will we make the computer figure this out? Another example could be to find the position of the person in the image to the right. How can we make the computer calculate this? The answer to both questions is twofold. First, we have to separate the different objects in the image and then we have to evaluate which object is the one we are looking for, i.e., circles and humans, respectively. The former process is known as BLOB extraction and the latter as BLOB classification. BLOB stands for Binary Large OBject and refers to a group of connected pixels in a binary image. The term "Large" indicates that only objects of a certain size are of interest and that "small" binary objects are usually noise.

The title of the chapter refers to analyzing binary images by first separating the BLOBs and secondly classifying the type of each BLOB based on their respective BLOB features. These topics will be described in more detail in the next sections.

In this chapter we work with binary images. A binary image is typically a result of applying some kind of threshold or classification algorithm to a gray level or color image. More information about thresholding and classification can be found in Chaps. 4 and 9.

7.1 BLOB Extraction

The purpose of BLOB extraction is to isolate the BLOBs (objects) in a binary image. As mentioned above, a BLOB consists of a group of connected pixels. Whether or not two pixels are connected is defined by the *connectivity*, that is, which pixels are neighbors and which are not. The two most often applied types of connectivity are illustrated in Fig. 7.2. The 8-connectivity is more accurate than the 4-connectivity, but the 4-connectivity is often applied since it requires fewer computations, hence

© Springer Nature Switzerland AG 2020
R. R. Paulsen and T. B. Moeslund, *Introduction to Medical Image Analysis*,
Undergraduate Topics in Computer Science,
https://doi.org/10.1007/978-3-030-39364-9_7

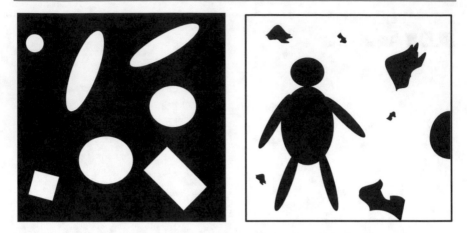

Fig. 7.1 A binary image containing different shapes and a binary image containing a human and some noise

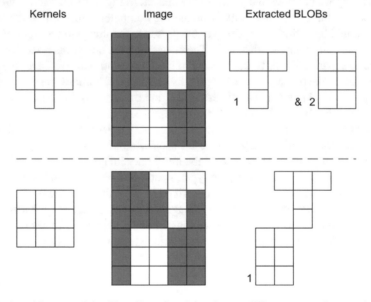

Fig. 7.2 4- and 8-connectivity. The effect of applying the two different types of connectivity

it can process the image faster. The effect of the two different types of connectivity is illustrated in Fig. 7.2 where the binary images contain either one or two BLOBs depending on the connectivity.

A number of different algorithms exist for finding the BLOBs and such algorithms are usually referred to as *connected component analysis* or *connected component labeling*. In the following, we describe one of these algorithms known as the *Grass-fire algorithm*. We use 4-connectivity for simplicity.

7.1.1 The Grass-Fire Algorithm

The algorithm starts in the upper-left corner of the binary image. It then scans the entire image from left to right and from top to bottom, as seen in Fig. 4.24.

At some point, during the scan an object pixel (white pixel) is encountered and the notion of grass-fire comes into play. In the binary image in Fig. 7.3 the first object pixel is found at the coordinate $(2, 0)$. At this point you should imagine yourself standing in a field covered with dry grass. Imagine you have four arms (!) and are holding a burning match in each hand. You then stretch out your arms in four different directions (corresponding to the neighbors in the 4-connectivity) and simultaneously drop the burning matches. When they hit the dry grass they will each start fire which again will spread in four new directions (up, down, left, right), etc. The result is that every single straw *which is connected* to your initial position will burn. This is the grass-fire principle. Note that if the grass field contains a river the grass on the other side will not be burned.

Returning to our binary image, the object pixels are the "dry grass" and the non-object pixels are water. So, the algorithm looks in four different directions and if it finds a pixel which can be "burned", meaning an object pixel, it does two things. Firstly, in the output image it gives this pixel an object label (basically a number) and secondly it "burns" the pixel in the input image by setting it to zero (black). Setting it to zero indicates that it has been burned and will therefore not be part of yet another fire. In the real grass field, the fire will spread simultaneously in all directions. In the computer, however, we can only perform one action at the time and the grass-fire is therefore performed as follows.

Let us apply the principle on Fig. 7.3. The pixel at the coordinate $(2, 0)$ is labeled 1, since it is the first BLOB and then burned (marked by a 1 in the lower right corner). Next, the algorithm tries to start a fire at the first neighbor $(3, 0)$, by checking if it is an object pixel or not. It is indeed an object pixel and is therefore labeled 1 (same object) and "burned". Since $(3, 0)$ is an object pixel, it now becomes the center of attention and its first neighbor is investigated $(4, 0)$. Again, this is an object pixel and is therefore labeled 1, "burned" and made center of attention. The first neighbor of $(4, 0)$ is outside the image and therefore per definition not an object pixel. The algorithm, therefore, investigates its second neighbor $(4, 1)$. This is not an object pixel and the third neighbor of $(4, 0)$ is therefore investigated $(3, 0)$. This has been burned and is therefore no longer an object pixel. Then the last neighbor of $(4, 0)$ is investigated $(4, -1)$. This is outside the image and therefore not an object pixel. All the neighbors of $(4, 0)$ have now been investigated and the algorithm, therefore, traces back and looks at the second neighbor of $(3, 0)$, namely, $(3, 1)$. This is an object pixel and is therefore labeled 1, burned, and becomes the new focus of attention. In this way the algorithm also finds $(3, 2)$ to be part of object 1 and finally ends by investigating the fourth neighbor of $(2, 0)$.

All pixels which are part of the top object have now been labeled with the same label 1 meaning that this BLOB has been segmented. The algorithm then moves on following the scan path in Fig. 4.24 until it meets the next object pixel $(1, 3)$, which is then labeled 2, and starts a new grass-fire. The result will be the image shown in

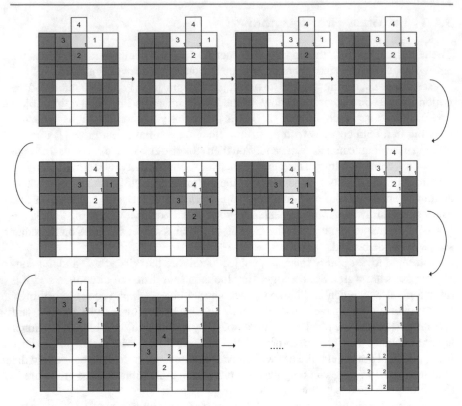

Fig. 7.3 The grass-fire algorithm. The "big" numbers indicate the order in which the neighbors are visited. The small numbers indicate the label of a pixel

Fig. 7.2, where each BLOB has a unique label. In Fig. 7.4 the BLOBs from Fig. 7.1 have been extracted and color coded according to their BLOB label. The result of applying a BLOB extraction algorithm to a binary image is therefore a label image.

7.2 BLOB Features

Extracting the BLOBs is the first step when confronted with examples like those presented in Fig. 7.1. The next step is to classify the different BLOBs. For the example with the circles, we want to classify each BLOB as either a circle or not a circle, and, for the other example, human versus non-human BLOBs. The classification process consists of two steps. First, each BLOB is represented by a number of characteristics, denoted *features*, and second, some matching method is applied to compare the features of each BLOB with the features of the type of object we are looking for. For example, to find circles we could calculate the circularity of each BLOB and

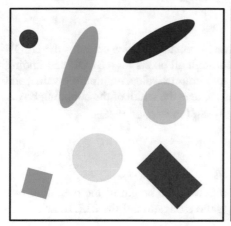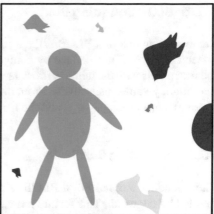

Fig. 7.4 Label images showing the BLOBs that were extracted from Fig. 7.1 using 4-connectivity. The BLOBs are color coded according to their label

compare that to the circularity of a perfect circle. Below we will first present how we can extract different features and then show how to compare features.

Feature extraction is a matter of converting each BLOB into a few representative numbers. That is, keep the relevant information and ignore the rest. But before calculating any features we first want to exclude every BLOB which is connected to the border of the image. The reason is that we in general have no information about the part of the object outside the image. For example, the semi-circle to the right of the human in Fig. 7.1 might look like a circle, but it might as well be the top of the head of a person lying down! Therefore, exclude all such BLOBs.

Having done so, a number of features can be calculated for each BLOB. Here follows a description of the most common features, but many others exist and new ones can be defined.

7.2.1   BLOB Area

The area of a BLOB is the number of pixels the BLOB consists of. This feature is often used to remove BLOBs that are too small or too big from the image. For example, in Fig. 7.1 (right) the human can be segmented by simply saying that all BLOBs with an area smaller than a certain value are ignored. Given a labeled image, the simplest way to find the area of a specific BLOB is to count all the pixels in the label image that has the label of the relevant BLOB.

7.2.2   BLOB Bounding Box

The bounding box of a BLOB is the minimum rectangle which contains the BLOB as seen in Fig. 7.5. It is defined by going through all pixels for a BLOB and finding the four pixels with the minimum x-value, maximum x-value, minimum y-value, and maximum y-value, respectively. From these values the width of the bounding box is given as $W_{BB} = x_{max} - x_{min}$ and the height as $H_{BB} = y_{max} - y_{min}$.

7.2.3   Bounding Box Ratio

The bounding box ratio of a BLOB is defined as the height of the bounding box divided by the width. This feature indicates the elongation of the BLOB, i.e., is the BLOB long, high, or neither.

7.2.4   Bounding Circle

of a BLOB is the minimum circle which contains the BLOB, see Fig. 7.5. It is found by first locating the center of the BLOB with one of the methods described below. Next we search from the center and outwards in one direction until we find the point where the BLOB ends. The distance between this point and the center is the radius in this direction. We do this for all possible directions (for example with an angular resolution of 10°) and the biggest radius defines the radius for the minimum circle.

7.2.5   Convex Hull

of a BLOB is the minimum convex polygon which contains the BLOB, see Fig. 7.5. It corresponds to placing a rubber band around the BLOB. It can be found in the following manner. From the topmost pixel on the BLOB search to the right along

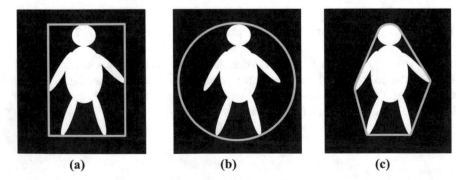

Fig. 7.5   a Bounding box. **b** Bounding circle. **c** Convex hull

a horizontal line. If no BLOB pixel is found, increase (clockwise) the angle of the search line and repeat the search. When a BLOB pixel is found, the first line of the polygon is defined and a new search is started based on the angle of the previous search line. When the search reappears at the topmost pixel, the convex hull is completed. Note that morphology also can be applied to find the convex hull of a BLOB.

7.2.6 Compactness

The compactness of a BLOB is defined as the ratio of the BLOB's area to the area of the bounding box. This can be used to distinguish compact BLOBs from non-compact ones. For example, fist versus a hand with outstretched fingers.

$$\text{Compactness} = \frac{\text{Area of BLOB}}{W_{BB} \cdot H_{BB}}, \tag{7.1}$$

where W_{BB} and H_{BB} are the height and width of the bounding box.

7.2.7 Center of Mass

The center of mass (or center of gravity or centroid) of a physical object is the location on the object where you should place your finger in order to balance the object. The center of mass for a binary image is similar. It is the average x- and y-positions of the binary object. It is defined as a point, whose x-value is calculated by summing the x-coordinates of all pixels in the BLOB and then dividing by the total number of pixels. Similarly for the y-value. In mathematical terms the center of mass, (x_c, y_c) is calculated as[1]:

$$x_c = \frac{1}{N} \sum_{i=1}^{N} x_i , \qquad y_c = \frac{1}{N} \sum_{i=1}^{N} y_i , \tag{7.2}$$

where N is the number of pixels in the BLOB and x_i and y_i are the x and y coordinates of the N pixels, respectively.

7.2.8 Perimeter

The perimeter of a BLOB is the length of the contour of the BLOB. This can be found by scanning along the rim (contour) of an object and summing the number of pixels encountered. A simple approximation of the perimeter is to first find the outer boundary using the method from Sect. 6.3.4 (or another edge detection algorithm). Following this, we simply count the number of white pixels in the image.

---

[1] See Appendix B for a definition of $\sum$.

7.2.9 Circularity

The circularity of a BLOB defines how circular a BLOB is. Different definitions exist based on the perimeter and area of the BLOB. Heywood's circularity factor is, for example, defined as the ratio of the BLOB's perimeter to the perimeter of the circle with the same area:

$$\text{Circularity} = \frac{\text{Perimeter of BLOB}}{2\sqrt{\pi} \cdot \text{Area of BLOB}} \ . \tag{7.3}$$

This circularity measure will have values in the range of $[1, \infty]$, where the value is 1 for the perfect circle and ∞ for a line. The circularity measure is based on that the area of a circle is given by $A = \pi r^2$, where r is the radius of the circle. The perimeter of a perfect circle is $P = 2\pi r$. Assume, we have found an object and can easily measure its area, A_m by counting pixels. If it is a perfect circle, the perimeter would then be $P_e = 2\sqrt{\pi A_m}$ (e means *estimated*). It is important that it is only for a perfectly circular object that P_e is actually the perimeter of the object—else it will always have a larger value. We have also measured the perimeter of the object, P_m, and by comparing it to P_e a measure of similarity can be given as Circularity $= P_m / P_e$ which is exactly the formula above. Sometimes the inverse of this measure is used:

$$\text{Circularity}_{\text{inverse}} = \frac{2\sqrt{\pi} \cdot \text{Area of BLOB}}{\text{Perimeter of BLOB}} \ . \tag{7.4}$$

This measure will be in the range of $[0, 1]$, where 1 is for the perfect circle and 0 for the line. Note that both Circularity and Circularity$_{\text{inverse}}$ can sometimes exceed the given intervals (Circularity being 0.97 for example). This is due to the estimation of the perimeter that is difficult to do exact.

In Fig. 7.6 four of the feature values are illustrated for the BLOBs in Fig. 7.1 (left). Note that it is the Circularity$_{\text{inverse}}$ that is used.

The features calculated for a single BLOB can now be collected in a *feature vector*. If we use the circularity and area features, then the feature vector for BLOB number one is

$$f_1 = \begin{bmatrix} 0.31 \\ 6561 \end{bmatrix} \ . \tag{7.5}$$

Since we have seven BLOBs, we will also have seven feature vectors: $f_1, \ldots, f_7$.

The number and types of feature that should be used are highly dependent on the objects that are in the images. In the following, a few methods to do this are explained.

7.3 BLOB Classification

BLOB classification means to put identified blobs into a set of classes, that are already defined. In the following examples, there are only two classes (circle versus not-circle) but the theory can also be applied when there are several different classes in the image. So in this example, we show how to determine which BLOB is a

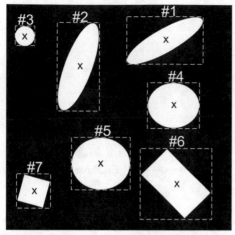

BLOB number	Circu-larity	Area (pixels)
1	0.31	6561
2	0.40	6544
3	0.98	890
4	0.97	6607
5	0.99	6730
6	0.52	6611
7	0.75	2073

Fig. 7.6 The Bounding Box and Center-of-Mass of each BLOB is seen to the left. To the right the Circularity$_{inverse}$ and Area for each BLOB is listed

circle and which is not. Each of the objects in Fig. 7.6 has been identified as separate BLOBs and a set of feature has been computed and put into feature vectors. As suggested above we can use the circularity feature for this purpose. In Fig. 7.6 the values of the circularity of the different BLOBs are listed. The question is now how to define which BLOBs are circles and which are not based on their feature values. For this purpose we make a *prototype model* of the object we are looking for. That is, what are the feature values of a perfect circle and what kind of deviations will we accept. In a perfect world we will not accept any deviations from the prototype, but in practice the object or the segmentation of the object will not be perfect so we have to accept some deviations. For our example with the circles, we can define the prototype to have a circularity of 1 and a deviation of ±0.15, meaning that BLOBs with circularity values in the range [0.85, 1.15] are accepted as circles. In general, the deviation needs to be defined with respect to the concrete application you are working with. Note also that the used circularity measure (Eq. 7.4) should not exceed that value of 1. Later it is shown how feature value ranges can be estimated using a set of training data.

The deviation results in a range, as seen above, when we only have one feature. In case of two features (with the same deviation) it defines a circle, three features result in a sphere, and more than three features result in a hypersphere. To illustrate this, let us reformulate the circle detection task to a matter of detecting only large circles. For this task one feature is not sufficient and we therefore use both the circularity and the area, see Fig. 7.6. These two features span a two-dimensional *feature space* as seen in Fig. 7.7. The prototype of a large circle is represented as "x" and the dashed circle around it represents the allowed deviation. So if a BLOB in an image has feature values inside the dashed circle, then it is classified as a large circle otherwise it is not.

Fig. 7.7 2D feature space
and position of the seven
BLOBs from Fig. 7.1 (left).
The "x" represents the
feature values of the
prototype and the dashed
circle illustrates the allowed
deviation. Note that neither
of the two features can
separate the large circles
from all other BLOBs

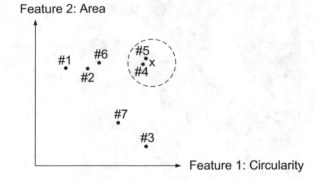

Whether or not the feature values of a BLOB are within the dashed circle is determined by calculating the Euclidean distance between the prototype and the BLOB in feature space. The feature vector of the model BLOB is

$$f_m = \begin{bmatrix} 1 \\ 6700 \end{bmatrix} . \tag{7.6}$$

The Euclidean distance in feature space between BLOB number one is, for example,

$$D = \sqrt{(0.31 - 1)^2 + (6561 - 6700)^2} . \tag{7.7}$$

This can be compactly written as $D = \| f_1 - f_m \|^2$, where $\|.\|$ is the *Euclidean norm*.

In this example, the area is measured in 1000s and the values of circularity are only around 0.30–1. This means that the distance in feature space, D, is completely dominated by the area value and that circularity has no influence. A solution is to do *feature normalization*, where all features will end up having values in the same interval [0, 1]. There are several different approaches to this. One approach is to first estimate the minimum and maximum values for each feature. In our example, it could be that we assume that the area minimum and maximum values are $A_{min} = 500$ and $A_{max} = 7000$ and for circularity $C_{min} = 0.25$ and $C_{max} = 1.1$. The normalized features will then become

$$\text{Area feature} = \frac{\text{Area} - A_{min}}{A_{max} - A_{min}} \tag{7.8}$$

$$\text{Circularity feature} = \frac{\text{Circularity} - C_{min}}{C_{max} - C_{min}} . \tag{7.9}$$

Another possible source of error is that the covariance of the features should be zero. This is beyond the scope of this book and the reader is referred to a text on multivariate statistics or pattern recognition.

7.4 Cell Classification Using BLOB Analysis

In this chapter, an example using cells is given to explain and demonstrate some important terms used in general object recognition and classification. The data are images from an instrument called an *image cytometer* produced by the Danish company Chemometec. The cells are fibroblast-like cell lines derived from monkey kidney tissue (COS-7). The goal of this example is to detect all cells with one cell nucleus. The cell nuclei can be seen to the right in Fig. 7.8, where a so-called DAPI staining has been used to make the nuclei visible in a fluorescence microscope. Other objects are also visible. For example, nuclei that are clumped together or undergoing transformations. The specific goal is to identify all single-nuclei and discard the remaining objects. In the following, a single-nucleus is just called *nucleus* (plural nuclei) and all other objects (including multiple clustered nuclei) are called *noise*. The classification will therefore be classifies into two classes: *nucleus* and *noise*.

7.4.1 Training Data

To be able to classify the nuclei a good approach is to *learn* the best features and the limits of the features values from *training data*. This data should be very similar to the data that should be classified. In Fig. 7.9, a part of the training data can be seen. The real training image is several times larger. The most important image is seen to the right where all nuclei has been marked. The marking was done by first setting a suitable threshold to create a binary image. After that a *morphological opening* was done followed by a *morphological closing* both using a circular structuring element of size 5×5. This was done to remove noise pixels and fill small holes in the objects. See Chap. 6 for information about *opening and closing*. Finally, all objects that are

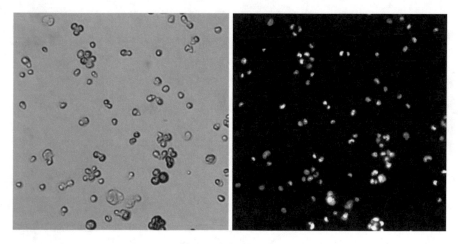

Fig. 7.8 COS-7 cell images taken with Chemometec image cytometer. In the left, the image is taken using ultraviolet microscopy and to the right fluorescence microscopy with DAPI staining

not nuclei were removed using an image editing tool. The result is an image with 439 well-defined nuclei. It is important that manual user annotation is not an error-free method and some annotations might be wrong.

7.4.2 Feature Selection and Feature Ranges

By looking at the images in Fig. 7.9, it is obvious that area and circularity could be good features to use when identifying good nuclei. There might be other good features but in the following we just use these two features. To see what we can learn from the training data, the two features are plotted against each other as seen in Fig. 7.10, where the histograms of the two features are also seen. In the plots, it can be clearly seen that there are some outliers in the annotated (manually marked) data. In this example, we use the plots to set the limits for the features that are used in future classification. This range selection can be done using statistical methods, but here they are just manually chosen. The feature value limits that are chosen are

Feature	Minimum	Maximum
Area	50	110
Circularity	0.87	1.05

These limits correspond to a rectangle in the feature space as seen in Fig. 7.9 (red rectangle). All objects that have features inside this rectangle will be classified as a nuclei. This is different from the previous example, where the region was made by a circle as seen in Fig. 7.7. By using the individual feature ranges, it is not necessary to compute a feature distance or worry about feature normalization. It can be seen

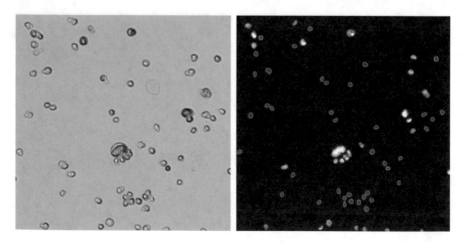

Fig. 7.9 Training images. To the left the UV microscopy image. To the right the DAPI stained image with manual annotations in red

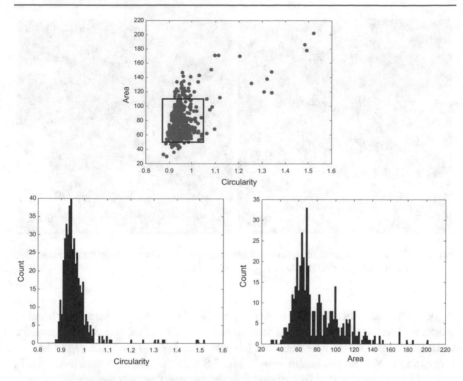

Fig. 7.10 Plots and histograms of the training data features for the cells seen in Fig. 7.9. The area is measured in pixels. The feature ranges are shown as a red rectangle

that these limits will classify some of our training samples to be *noise* but this can be due to the fact that it is difficult to do hundred percent correct manual annotation. Later, the consequence of setting the feature range limits will be investigated.

Now our algorithm is ready. To sum it up, it takes image and creates a binary image by using a threshold. After that a *morphological opening* is done followed by a *morphological closing* both using a circular structuring element of size 5×5. Now all the BLOBs are found and the BLOBs touching the border of the image are removed. For each BLOB the area and circularity are computed and compared to the rectangle from Fig. 7.10. Then the BLOBs inside the rectangle are classified as *nuclei* and the ones outside as *noise*. So we are now ready to classify objects on new and unseen images. However, it is important first to get an idea of how good our classification algorithm is.

7.4.3   Evaluation of Classification

It is important to find out how well a classifier performs. One option is to see how well it classifies the objects in the images used for training. However, this is a not

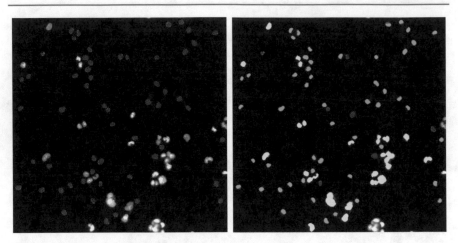

Fig. 7.11 To the left is the ground truth annotation and to the right is the classification result. True positives: green, false positive: red, false negatives: blue and true negatives: yellow

a good approach since there is a very high risk of *overfitting*, where the classifier works well on the training data but fails on new data. The usual approach is therefore to test the classifier on new data that has not been used to train the algorithm. In this example, we use the image seen in Fig. 7.8 with the nuclei annotations seen in Fig. 7.11 as *ground-truth*. This means that we assume that that the marked objects are *true nuclei* and all other objects are *noise*.

The classification algorithm that was developed is now run on the ground truth image and the result of the classification is compared to the ground truth. In the following, a *confusion matrix* is used to describe how good our classification algorithm is. Lets first look at our *ground truth image* where there are in total $N = 77$ objects. Of these, 56 are marked as being *nuclei* we call them for *actual positives* and the other 21 objects (*noise*) for *actual negatives*. The goal is that our classifier is as good as possible in correctly predicting the positives and the negatives. When comparing the objects classified with the algorithm and the ground truth there are the following possibilities:

True Positive (TP) A *nuclei* is classified as a *nuclei*
True Negative (TN) A *noise object* is classified as *noise object*
False Positive (FP) A *noise object* is classified as a *nuclei*
False Negative (FN) A *nuclei* is classified as a *noise object*.

These four cases are shown in Fig. 7.11 to the right, where they are colored as TP = green, TN = yellow, FP = red, FN = blue. The values can now be combined into the *confusion matrix*, where the values come from our example seen in Fig. 7.11:

The numbers seen in the confusion matrix can be combined into a set of rates, that all describe the performance of the classifier:

	Predicted as noise	Predicted as single-nuclei
Actual Noise	TN = 19	FP = 2
Actual single-nuclei	FN = 5	TP = 51

Accuracy Tells how often the classifier is correct: (TP + TN)/N.

Misclassification rate How often is the classifier wrong: (FP + FN)/N.

True positive rate How often is a positive predicted when it actually is positive: TP/(FN + TP). Also called *sensitivity*.

False positive rate How often is a positive predicted when it actually is negative: FP/(TN + FP).

Specificity How often is a negative predicted when it actually is negative: TN/(TN + FP).

Precision How often is it correct when a positive is predicted: TP/(FP + TP).

In the example the accuracy is $(51 + 19)/77 = 91\%$ and the misclassification rate is $(2 + 5)/77 = 9\%$. The true positive rate is $51/(5 + 51) = 91\%$ and the false positive rate is $2/(19 + 2) = 10\%$.

It is very dependent on the actual problem to decide if the performance of an algorithm is acceptable. In this case, where the identification of single-nuclei is used for further processing of the cell, it is not critical that a few nuclei are not detected. However, it would be bad if a noise object was identified as a nuclei and used in the further analysis. So in this case it would be better to have a very low *false positive rate* than having a high *true positive rate*. For cancer diagnostic (here positive means having cancer) it would probably be better to have a very high *true positive rate* to not miss any potential tumors even if it means an increase *false positive rate* as well. The classification rates can be optimized by changing the feature ranges and thereby changing the shape of the rectangle in Fig. 7.10. It is important to remember that every time the values are changed the algorithm should be tested on a fresh set of evaluation images to avoid overfitting.

Color Images

8

So far we have restricted ourselves to gray-scale images, but, as you might have noticed, the real world consists of colors. Going back some years, many cameras (and displays, e.g., TV monitors) only handled gray-scale images. As the technology matured, it became possible to capture (and visualize) color images and today most cameras can capture color images.

In this chapter, we turn to the topic of color images. We describe the nature of color images and how they are captured and represented, before expanding one of the methods from the previous chapters to also include color images.

8.1 What Is a Color?

In Chap. 2 it was explained that an image is formed by measuring the amount of energy entering the image sensor. It was also stated that only energy within a certain frequency/wavelength range is measured. This wavelength range is denoted the *visual spectrum*. In the human eye, this is done by the so-called *rods*, which are specialized nerve cells that act as *photoreceptors*. Besides the rods, the human eye also contains *cones*. These operate like the rods, but are not sensitive to all wavelengths in the visual spectrum. Instead, the eye contains three types of cones, each sensitive to different wavelength ranges. The human brain interprets the output from these different cones as different colors as seen in Table 8.1 [1].

So, a color is defined by a certain wavelength in the electromagnetic spectrum as illustrated in Fig. 8.1. Due to the three different types of cones we have the notion of the *primary colors* being red, green, and blue. Psycho-visual experiments have shown that the different cones have different sensitivity. This means that when you see two different colors with the same intensity, you will judge their brightness differently. On average, a human perceives red as being 2.6 times as bright as blue and green as

© Springer Nature Switzerland AG 2020
R. R. Paulsen and T. B. Moeslund, *Introduction to Medical Image Analysis*,
Undergraduate Topics in Computer Science,
https://doi.org/10.1007/978-3-030-39364-9_8

Table 8.1 The different types of photoreceptors in the human eye. The cones are each specialized to a certain wavelength range and peak response within the visual spectrum. The output from each of the three types of cones is interpreted as a particular color by the human brain: red, green, and blue, respectively. The rods measure the amount of energy in the visual spectrum, hence the shade of gray. The type indicators L,M,S, are short for long, medium, and short, respectively, and refer to the wavelength

Photoreceptor cell	Wavelength in nanometers (nm)	Peak response in nanometer (nm)	Interpretation by the human brain
Cones (type L)	[400–680]	564	Red
Cones (type M)	[400–650]	534	Green
Cones (type S)	[370–530]	420	Blue
Rods	[400–600]	498	Shade of gray

Fig. 8.1 The relationship between colors and wavelengths

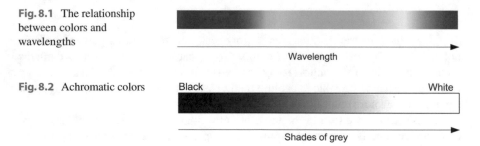

Wavelength

Fig. 8.2 Achromatic colors

Black   White

Shades of grey

being 5.6 times as bright as blue. Hence, the eye is more sensitive to green and least sensitive to blue.

When all wavelengths (all colors) are present at the same time, the eye perceives this as a shade of gray, hence no color is seen! If the energy level increases, the shade becomes brighter and ultimately becomes white. Conversely, when the energy level is decreased, the shade becomes darker and ultimately becomes black. This continuum of different gray-levels (or shades of gray) is denoted the *achromatic colors* and illustrated in Fig. 8.2. Note that this is the same as Fig. 2.18.

An image is created by sampling the incoming light. The colors of the incoming light depend on the color of the light source illuminating the scene and the material the object is made of, see Fig. 8.3. Some of the light that hits the object will bounce right off and some will penetrate into the object. An amount of this light will be absorbed by the object and an amount leaves again possibly with a different color. So when you see a green car this means that the wavelengths of the main light reflected from the car are in the range of the type M cones, see Table 8.1. If we assume the car was illuminated by the sun, which emits all wavelengths, then we can reason that all wavelengths *except* the green ones are absorbed by the material the car is made of. Or in other words, if you are wearing a black shirt all wavelengths (energy) are absorbed by the shirt and this is why it becomes hotter than a white shirt.

Fig. 8.3 The different
components influencing the
color of the received light

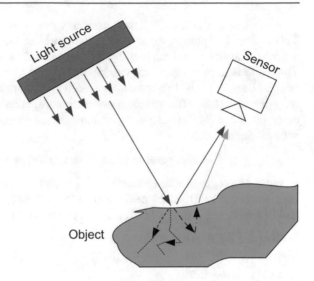

When the resulting color is created by illuminating an object by white light and
then absorbing some of the wavelengths (colors) we use the notion of *subtractive
colors*. Exactly as when you mix paint to create a color. Say you start with a white
piece of paper, where no light is absorbed. The resulting color will be white. If you
then want the paper to become green you add green paint, which absorbs everything
but the green wavelengths. If you add yet another color of paint, then more wavelengths will be absorbed, and hence the resulting light will have a new color. Keep
doing this and you will, in theory, end up with a mixture where all wavelengths are
absorbed, that is, black. In practice, however, it will probably not be black, but rather
dark gray/brown.

The opposite of subtractive colors is *additive colors*. This notion applies when you
create the wavelengths as opposed to manipulating white light. A good example is a
color monitor like a computer screen or a TV screen. Here each pixel is a combination
of emitted red, green, and blue light. Meaning that a black pixel is generated by not
emitting anything at all. White (or rather a shade of gray) is generated by emitting
the same amount of red, green, and blue. Red will be created by only emitting red
light etc. All other colors are created by a combination of red, green, and blue. For
example, yellow is created by emitting the same amount of red and green, and no
blue.

8.2 Representation of an RGB Color Image

A color camera is based on the same principle as the human eye. That is, it measures
the amount of incoming red light, green light, and blue light, respectively. This is
done in one of two ways depending on the number of sensors in the camera. In the

case of three sensors, each sensor measures one of the three colors, respectively. This is done by splitting the incoming light into the three wavelength ranges using some optical filters and mirrors. So red light is only send to the "red-sensor", etc. The result is three images each describing the amount of red, green, and blue light per pixel, respectively. In a color image, each pixel therefore consists of three values: red, green, and blue. The actual representation might be three images—one for each color, but it can also be a three-dimensional vector for each pixel, hence an image of vectors. Such a vector looks like this[1]:

$$\text{Color pixel} = [\text{Red, Green, Blue}] = [R, G, B] \ . \tag{8.1}$$

In terms of programming a color pixel is usually represented as a *struct*. Say we want to set the RGB values of the pixel at position $(2, 4)$ to: Red=100, Green=42, and Blue=10, respectively. In C-code this can be written as

Setting the RGB value

```
f[2][4].R = 100;
f[2][4].G = 42;
f[2][4].B = 10;
```

respectively; or alternatively:

Setting the RGB value

```
SetPixel(image, 2, 4, R, 100);
SetPixel(image, 2, 4, G, 42);
SetPixel(image, 2, 4, B, 10);
```

Typically each color value is represented by an 8-bit (one byte) value meaning that 256 different shades of each color can be measured. Combining different values of the three colors, each pixel can represent $256^3 = 16, 777, 216$ different colors.

A cheaper alternative to having three sensors including mirrors and optical filters is to only have one sensor. In this case, each cell in the sensor is made sensitive to one of the three colors (ranges of wavelengths). This can be done in a number of different ways. One is using a *Bayer pattern*. Here 50% of the cells are sensitive to green, while the remaining cells are divided equally between red and blue. The reason being, as mentioned above, that the human eye is more sensitive to green. The layout of the different cells is illustrated in Fig. 8.4 to the left.

The figure shows the upper-left corner of the sensor, where the letters illustrate which color a particular pixel is sensitive to. This means that each pixel only captures one color and that the two other colors of a particular pixel must be inferred from the neighbors. Algorithms for finding the remaining colors of a pixel are known as *demosaicing* and, generally speaking, the algorithms are characterized by the

---

[1]See Appendix B for a definition of a vector.

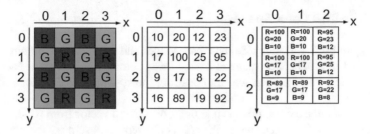

Fig. 8.4 Left: The Bayer pattern used for capturing a color image on a single image sensor. R = red, G = green, and B = blue. Middle: Numbers measured by the sensor. Right: Estimated RGB image using Eq. 8.2

required processing time (often directly proportional to the number of neighbors included) and the quality of the output. The higher the processing time the better the result. How to balance these two issues is up to the camera manufactures, and in general, the higher the quality of the camera, the higher the cost. Even very advanced algorithms are not as good as a three-sensor color camera and note that when using, for example, a cheap web-camera, the quality of the colors might not be too good and care should be taken before using the colors for any processing. Regardless of the choice of demosaicing algorithm, the output is the same as when using three sensors, namely, Eq. 8.1. That is, even though only one color is measured per pixel, the output for each pixel will (after demosaicing) consist of three values: R, G, and B.

An example of a simple demosaicing algorithm is to infer the missing colors from the nearest pixels, for example, using the following sets of equation:

$$g(x, y) \begin{cases} [R, G, B]_B & = [f(x + 1, y + 1), f(x + 1, y), f(x, y)] \\ [R, G, B]_{GB} = [f(x, y + 1), f(x, y), f(x - 1, y)] \\ [R, G, B]_{GR} = [f(x + 1, y), f(x, y), f(x, y - 1)] \\ [R, G, B]_R & = [f(x, y), f(x - 1, y), f(x - 1, y - 1)] \end{cases}, \qquad (8.2)$$

where $f(x, y)$ is the input image (Bayer pattern) and $g(x, y)$ is the output RGB image. The RGB values in the output image are found differently depending on which color a particular pixel is sensitive to: $[R, G, B]_B$ should be used for the pixels sensitive to blue, $[R, G, B]_R$ should be used for the pixels sensitive to red, and $[R, G, B]_{GB}$ and $[R, G, B]_{GR}$ should be used for the pixels sensitive to green followed by a blue or red pixel, respectively. In Fig. 8.4 a concrete example of this algorithm is illustrated. In the middle figure the values sampled from the sensor are shown. In the right figure the resulting RGB output image is shown using Eq. 8.2.

8.2.1   The RGB Color Space

According to Eq. 8.1 a color pixel has three values and can therefore be represented as one point in a 3D space spanned by the three colors. If we say that each color is represented by 8-bits, then we can construct the so-called RGB color cube, see Fig. 8.5.

In the color cube a color pixel is one point or rather a vector from (0, 0, 0) to the pixel value. The different corners in the color cube represent some of the *pure colors* and are listed in Table 8.2. The vector from (0, 0, 0) to (255, 255, 255) passes through all the gray-scale values and is denoted the *gray-vector*. Note that the gray-vector is identical to Fig. 8.2.

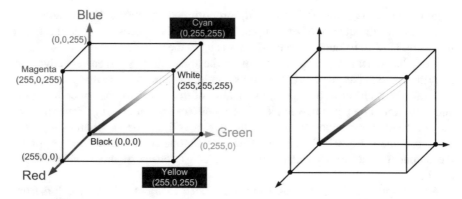

Fig. 8.5 Left: The RGB color cube. Right: The gray-vector in the RGB color cube

Table 8.2 The colors of the different corners in the RGB color cube

Corner	Color	
(0,0,0)	Black	
(255,0,0)	Red	
(0,255,0)	Green	
(0,0,255)	Blue	
(255,255,0)	Yellow	
(255,0,255)	Magenta	
(0,255,255)	Cyan	
(255,255,255)	White	

8.2.2   Converting from RGB to Gray-Scale

Even though you use a color camera it might be sufficient for your algorithm to apply the intensity information in the image and you therefore need to convert the color image into a gray-scale image. Converting from RGB to gray-scale is performed as:

$$I = W_R \cdot R + W_G \cdot G + W_B \cdot B \ , \tag{8.3}$$

where I is the intensity and $W_R + W_G + W_B = 1$ are weight factors for R, G, and B, respectively. As default the three colors are equally important, hence $W_R = W_G = W_B = \frac{1}{3}$, but depending on the application one or two colors might be more important and the weight factors should be set accordingly. For example, when processing images of vegetation the green color typically contains the most information or when processing images of metal objects the most information is typically located in the blue pixels. Yet another example could be when looking for human skin (face and hands) which has a reddish color. In general, the weights should be set according to your application and a good way of assessing this is by looking at the histograms of each color.

When the goal of a conversion from color to gray-scale is not to prepare the image for processing but rather for visualization purposes, then an understanding of the human visual perception can help decide the weight factors. The optimal weights vary from individual to individual, but the weights listed below are a good compromise, agreed upon by major international standardization organizations within TV and image/video coding. When the weights are optimized for the human visual system, the resulting gray-scale value is denoted *luminance* and usually represented as Y.

$$W_R = 0.299 \quad W_G = 0.587 \quad W_B = 0.114 \tag{8.4}$$

An example of a color image transformed into a gray-scale image using the luminance-based conversion can be seen in Fig. 8.6. Generally, it is not possible to convert a gray-scale image back into the original color image, since the color information is lost during the color to gray-scale transformation.

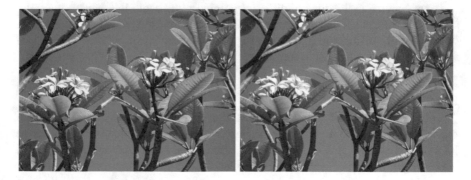

Fig. 8.6 Color to gray-scale conversion

Fig. 8.7 The RGB color cube. Each dot corresponds to a particular pixel value. Multiple dots on the same line all have the same color, but different levels of illumination

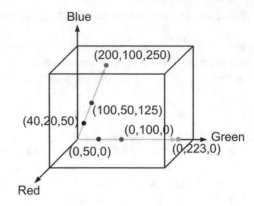

Fig. 8.8 Left: The triangle where all color vectors pass through. The value of a point on the triangle is defined using normalized RGB coordinates. Right: The chromaticity plane

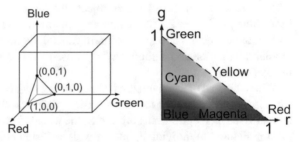

8.2.3   The Normalized RGB Color Representation

If we have the following three RGB pixel values (0,50,0), (0,100,0), and (0,223,0) in the RGB color cube, we can see that they all lie on the same vector, namely, the one spanned by (0,0,0) and (0,255,0). We say that all values are a shade of green and go even further and say that they all have the same color (green), but different levels of illumination. This also applies to the rest of the color cube. For example, the points (20,240,44), (10,120,22), and (5,60,11) all lie on the same vector and therefore have the same color, but just different illumination levels. This is illustrated in Fig. 8.7.

If we generalize this idea of different points on the same line having the same color, then we can see that all possible lines pass through the triangle defined by the points (1,0,0), (0,1,0), and (0,0,1), see Fig. 8.8 left. The actual point (r, g, b) where a line intersects the triangle is found as[2]:

$$(r, g, b) = \left(\frac{R}{R + G + B}, \frac{G}{R + G + B}, \frac{B}{R + G + B} \right) . \qquad (8.5)$$

These values are named *normalized RGB* and denoted (r, g, b). In Table 8.3 the rgb values of some RGB values are shown. Note that each value is in the interval [0, 1] and that $r + g + b = 1$. This means that if we know two of the normalized

---

[2]Note that the formula is undefined for $(R, G, B) = (0, 0, 0)$. We therefore make the following definition: $(r, g, b) \equiv (0, 0, 0)$ when $(R, G, B) = (0, 0, 0)$.

RGB values, then we can easily find the remaining value, or in other words, we can represent a normalized RGB color using just two of the values. Say we choose r and g, then this corresponds to representing the triangle in Fig. 8.8 left by the triangle to the right, see Fig. 8.8. This triangle is denoted the *chromaticity plane* and the colors along the edges of the triangle are the so-called pure colors. The further away from the edges the less pure the color and ultimately the center of the triangle has no color at all and is a shade of gray. It can be stated that the closer to the center a color is, the more "polluted" a pure color is by white light.

Summing up we can now re-represent an RGB value by its "*true*" color, r and g, and the amount of light (intensity or energy or illumination) in the pixel. That is

$$(R, G, B) \Leftrightarrow (r, g, I) , \tag{8.6}$$

where $I = \frac{R+G+B}{3}$. In Table 8.3 the rgI values of some RGB values are shown. Separating the color and the intensity like this can be a powerful notion in many applications. In Sect. 8.4 one will be presented.

In terms of programming the conversion from (R, G, B) to (r, g, I) can be implemented in C-Code as illustrated below:

Conversion from RGB to rgI

```
for (y = 0; y < M; y = y+1)
{
    for (x = 0; x < N; x = x+1)
    {
        temp =  GetPixel(input, x, y, R) +
                GetPixel(input, x, y, G) +
                GetPixel(input, x, y, B);
        value = GetPixel(input, x, y, R) / temp;
        SetPixel(output, x, y, r, value);
        value = GetPixel(input, x, y, G) / temp;
        SetPixel(output, x, y, g, value);
        value = temp / 3;
        SetPixel(output, x, y, I, value);
    }
}
```

Here M is the height of the image, N is the width of the image, input is the RGB image, and output is the rgI image. The programming example primarily consists of two *FOR-loops* which go through the image, pixel-by-pixel, and convert from an input image (RGB) to an output image (rgI). The opposite conversion from (r, g, I) to (R, G, B) can be implemented as

Table 8.3 Some different colors and their representation in the different color spaces. ND = Not Defined

Color	(R,G,B)	(r,g,b)	(r,g,I)	(H,S,I)
Red	(255,0,0)	(1,0,0)	(1,0,85)	(0,1,85)
Yellow	(255,255,0)	(1/2,1/2,0)	(1/2,1/2,170)	(60,1,170)
Green	(0,255,0)	(0,1,0)	(0,1,85)	(120,1,85)
Cyan	(0,255,255)	(0,1/2,1/2)	(0,1/2,170)	(180,1,170)
Blue	(0,0,255)	(0,0,1)	(0,0,85)	(240,1,85)
Magenta	(255,0,255)	(1/2,0,1/2)	(1/2,0,170)	(300,1,170)
Black	(0,0,0)	(0,0,0)	(0,0,0)	(ND,0,0)
White	(255,255,255)	(1/3,1/3,1/3)	(1/3,1/3,255)	(ND,0,255)
25% white	(64,64,64)	(1/3,1/3,1/3)	(1/3,1/3,64)	(ND,0,64)
50% white	(128,128,128)	(1/3,1/3,1/3)	(1/3,1/3,128)	(ND,0,128)
25% Blue	(0,0,64)	(0,0,1)	(0,0,21)	(240,1,21)
50% Blue	(0,0,128)	(0,0,1)	(0,0,43)	(240,1,43)
75% Blue	(0,0,192)	(0,0,1)	(0,0,64)	(240,1,64)
Orange	(255,165,0)	(0.6,0.4,0)	(0.6,0.4,140)	(40,1,140)
Pink	(255,192,203)	(0.4,0.3,0.3)	(0.4,0.3,217)	(351,0.1,217)
Brown	(165,42,42)	(0.6,0.2,0.2)	(0.6,0.2,83)	(0,0.5,83)

Conversion from rgI to RGB

```
for (y = 0; y < M; y = y+1)
{
    for (x = 0; x < N; x = x+1)
    {
        temp = 3 * GetPixel(input,x,y,I);
        value = GetPixel(input, x, y, r) * temp;
        SetPixel(output, x, y, R, value);
        value = GetPixel(input, x, y, g) * temp;
        SetPixel(output, x, y, G, value);
        value = (1 - GetPixel(input, x, y, r) -
                GetPixel(input, x, y, g)) * temp;
        SetPixel(output, x, y, B, value);
    }
}
```

Here `input` is the rgI image, and `output` is the RGB image.

8.3 Other Color Representations

From a human perception point of view, the triangular representation in Fig. 8.8b is not intuitive. Instead humans rather use the notion of *hue* and *saturation*, when perceiving colors. The hue is the dominant wavelength in the perceived light and represents the pure color, i.e., the colors located on the edges of the triangle in Fig. 8.8b. The saturation is the purity of the color and represents the amount of white light mixed with the pure color. To understand these entities better, let us look at Fig. 8.9 left. First of all, we see that the point C corresponds to the neutral point, meaning the colorless center of the triangle, where $(r, g) = (1/3, 1/3)$. Let us define a random point in the triangle as P. The hue of this point is now defined as an angle, θ, between the vectors $\overrightarrow{Cr}$ and $\overrightarrow{CP}$. So hue $= 0°$ means red and hue $= 120°$ means green.

If the point P is located on the edge of the triangle then we say the saturation is 1, hence a pure color. As the point approaches C the saturation goes towards 0, and ultimately becomes 0 when $P = C$. Since the distance from C to the three edges of the triangle is not uniform, the saturation is defined as a relative distance. That is, saturation is defined as the ratio between the distance from C to P, and the distance from C to the point on the edge of the triangle in the direction of $\overrightarrow{CP}$. Mathematically we have

$$\text{Saturation} = \frac{\|\overrightarrow{CP}\|}{\|\overrightarrow{CP'}\|} \qquad \text{Hue} = \theta \ , \qquad\qquad (8.7)$$

where $\|\overrightarrow{CP}\|$ is the length of the vector $\overrightarrow{CP}$, see Appendix B. The representation of colors based on hue and saturation results in a circle as opposed to the triangle in Fig. 8.8 right. In Fig. 8.9 right the hue-saturation representation is illustrated together with some of the pure colors. It is important to realize how this figure relates to Fig. 8.5, or in other words, how the hue-saturation representation relates to the RGB representation. The center of the hue-saturation circle in Fig. 8.9 right is a shade of gray and corresponds to the gray-vector in Fig. 8.5. The circle is located so that it is perpendicular to the gray-vector. For a particular RGB value, the hue-saturation circle is therefore centered at a position on the gray-vector, so that the RGB value is included in the circle.

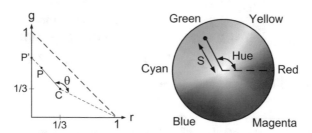

Fig. 8.9 Left: The definition of hue and saturation. Right: The hue-saturation representation. The color of a pixel (indicated by a dot) is represented by a hue value and a saturation value (denoted S in the figure). The figure also indicates the location of some of the pure colors

A number of different color representations exist, which are based on the notion of hue and saturation. Below one of these is presented.[3]

8.3.1   The HSI Color Representation

The HSI color representation is short for hue, saturation, and intensity. The representation follows the exact definition mentioned above. That is, the intensity is defined as $I = \frac{R+G+B}{3}$ and hue and saturation is defined as illustrated in Fig. 8.9. When calculating the conversion from RGB to HSI we seek a way of avoiding first converting from RGB to rg, i.e., we want to represent the conversion in terms of RGB values. It can be shown that the resulting conversion from RGB to HSI is defined as [5]:

$$H = \begin{cases} \cos^{-1}\left(1/2 \cdot \frac{(R-G)+(R-B)}{\sqrt{(R-G)(R-G)+(R-B)(G-B)}}\right), & \text{if } G \geq B; \\ 360° - \cos^{-1}\left(1/2 \cdot \frac{(R-G)+(R-B)}{\sqrt{(R-G)(R-G)+(R-B)(G-B)}}\right), & \text{Otherwise.} \end{cases} \tag{8.8}$$

$$H \in [0, 360[$$

$$S = 1 - 3 \cdot \frac{\min\{R, G, B\}}{R + G + B} \qquad S \in [0, 1] \tag{8.9}$$

$$I = \frac{R + G + B}{3} \qquad I \in [0, 255] , \tag{8.10}$$

where $\min\{R, G, B\}$ means the smallest of the R, G, and B values, see Appendix B. Saturation is defined to be zero when $(R, G, B) = (0, 0, 0)$ and hue is undefined for gray-values, i.e., when $R = G = B$. The conversion from HSI to RGB is given as

$$H_n = \begin{cases} 0, & \text{if } 0° \leq H \leq 120°; \\ H - 120°, & \text{if } 120° < H \leq 240°; \\ H - 240°, & \text{if } 240° < H < 360°; \end{cases} \tag{8.11}$$

$$R = \begin{cases} I \cdot \left(1 + \frac{S \cdot \cos(H_n)}{\cos(60° - H_n)}\right), & \text{if } 0° \leq H \leq 120°; \\ I - I \cdot S, & \text{if } 120° < H \leq 240°; \\ 3I - G - B, & \text{if } 240° < H < 360°; \end{cases} \tag{8.12}$$

$$G = \begin{cases} 3I - R - B, & \text{if } 0° \leq H \leq 120°; \\ I \cdot \left(1 + \frac{S \cdot \cos(H_n)}{\cos(60° - H_n)}\right), & \text{if } 120° < H \leq 240°; \\ I - I \cdot S, & \text{if } 240° < H < 360°; \end{cases} \tag{8.13}$$

$$B = \begin{cases} I - I \cdot S, & \text{if } 0° \leq H \leq 120°; \\ 3I - R - G, & \text{if } 120° < H \leq 240°; \\ I \cdot \left(1 + \frac{S \cdot \cos(H_n)}{\cos(60° - H_n)}\right), & \text{if } 240° < H < 360°; \end{cases} \tag{8.14}$$

In Table 8.3 the HSI values of some RGB pixels are shown.[4]

---

[3] It should be noted that the naming of the different color representations based on hue and saturation is not consistent throughout the body of literature covering this subject. Please have this in mind when studying other information sources.

[4] Note that sometimes all parameters are normalized to the interval [0, 1]. For example for H this is done as $H_{\text{normalized}} = \frac{H}{360}$.

8.4   Color Thresholding

Color thresholding can be a powerful approach to segmenting objects in a scene. Imagine you want to detect the hands of a human for controlling some interface. This can be done in a number of ways, where the easiest might be to ask the user to wear colored gloves. If this is combined with the restriction that the particular color of the gloves is neither present in the background nor on the rest of the user, then by finding all pixels with the color of the gloves we have found the hands. This operates similarly to the thresholding operation described in Eq. 4.20. The difference is that each of the color values of a pixel is compared to two threshold values, i.e., in total six threshold values. If each color value for a pixel is within the threshold values, then the pixel is set to white (foreground pixel) otherwise black (background pixel). The algorithm looks as follows for each pixel:

$$
\begin{aligned}
&\textbf{If}\\
&\quad R > R_{min} \quad \text{and} \quad R < R_{max} \quad \text{and}\\
&\quad G > G_{min} \quad \text{and} \quad G < G_{max} \quad \text{and}\\
&\quad B > B_{min} \quad \text{and} \quad B < B_{max}\\
&\textbf{Then} \quad g(x, y) = 255\\
&\textbf{Else} \quad\ \ g(x, y) = 0,
\end{aligned}
\tag{8.15}
$$

where (R, G, B) are the RGB values of the pixel being processed and R_{min} and R_{max} define the range of acceptable values of red in order to accept the current pixel as belonging to an object of interest (similarly for green and blue).

The algorithm actually corresponds to defining a box in the RGB color cube space and classifying a pixel as belonging to an object if it is within the box and otherwise classifying it as background. This is illustrated in Fig. 8.10.

One problem with color thresholding is its sensitivity to changes in the illumination. Say you have defined your threshold values so that the system can detect the two gloved hands. If someone increases the amount of light in the room, the color will stay the same, but the intensity will change. To handle such a situation, you need to increase/decrease the threshold values accordingly. This will result in the box in Fig. 8.10 being larger and hence the risk of including non-glove pixels will increase. In the worst case, the box will be as large as the entire RGB color cube.

Fig. 8.10 The box is defined by the threshold values. The box indicates the region within the RGB color cube where object pixels lie

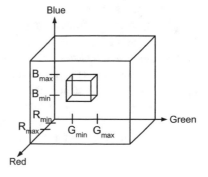

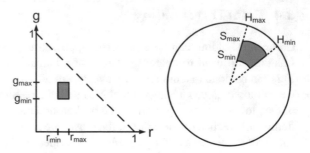

Fig. 8.11 The two gray shapes are defined by threshold values and indicate the regions within the two color spaces where object pixels lie. Left: The rg-color space. Right: The hs-color space

The solution is to convert the RGB color image into a representation where the color and intensity are separated, and then do color thresholding on only the colors, e.g., rg-values or hs-values. The thresholds can now be tighter, hence reducing the risk of false classification. In Fig. 8.11 the equivalent of Fig. 8.10 is shown for rg- and hs-representations, respectively. Regardless of which color representation is applied, the problem of choosing proper threshold values is the same.

Note that some thresholding on the intensity values is often a good idea. If you look at the color cube you can see that all possible colors will have a vector starting in $(0, 0, 0)$. This means that the vectors will lie in the vicinity of $(0, 0, 0)$ and the practical meaning of this is that it is hard to distinguish colors when the intensity is low. Therefore, it is often a good idea not to process the colors of pixels with low intensity values. Like, color pixels with a very high intensity might also be problematic to process. Say we have a pixel with the following RGB values $(255, 250, 250)$. This will be interpreted as very close to white and hence containing no color. But it might be that the real values are $(10000, 250, 250)$. You have no way of knowing, since the red value is saturated in the image acquisition process. So the red pixel is incorrectly classified as (close to) white. In general, you should try to avoid saturated pixels in the image acquisition process, but when you do encounter them, please take great care before using the color of such a pixel. In fact, you are virtually always better off ignoring such pixels.

8.4.1 Chroma-Keying

A very popular use of color thresholding is to segment objects (especially people) by placing them in front of a unique colored background. The object pixels are then found as those pixels in the image, which do *not* have this unique color. This principle is denoted *chroma-keying* and used for special effects in many Hollywood productions as well as in TV weather forecasts, etc. In the latter example, the host appears to be standing in front of a weather map. In reality, the host is standing in front of a green or blue screen and the background pixels are then replaced by pixels from the weather map. Obviously, this only works when the color of the host's clothing is different from the unique color used for covering the background.

8.5   Postscript on Colors

When reading literature on color spaces and color processing it is important to realize that a number of different terms are used.[5] Unfortunately, some of these terms are used interchangeably even though they might have different physical/perceptual/technical meanings. We therefore give a guideline to some of the terms you are likely to encounter when reading different literature on colors:

Chromatic Color	All colors in the RGB color cube except those lying on the gray-line spanned by $(0, 0, 0)$ and $(255, 255, 255)$.
Achromatic Color	The colorless values in the RGB cube, i.e., all those colors lying on the gray-line. The opposite of chromatic color.
Shades of gray	The same as achromatic color.
Intensity	The average amount of energy, i.e., $(R + G + B)/3$
Brightness	The amount of light perceived by a human.
Lightness	The amount of light perceived by a human.
Luminance	The amount of light perceived by a human. Note that when you venture into the science of color understanding, the luminance defines the amount of emitted light.
Luma	Gamma-corrected luminance.
Shade	Darkening a color. When a subtractive color space is applied, different shades (darker nuances) of a color are obtained by mixing the color with different amounts of black.
Tint	Lightening a color. When a subtractive color space is applied, different tints (lighter nuances) of a color are obtained by mixing the color with different amounts of white.
Tone	A combination of shade and tint, where gray is mixed with the input color.
' (denoted prime)	The primed version of a color, i.e., R', means that the value has been gamma-corrected.

---

[5]When going into color perception and color understanding even more terms are added to the vocabulary.

Pixel Classification

9

Classification is an important tool in medical image analysis and is used for a variety of different diagnostics systems. In this chapter, we will focus on a special type of classification, dealing with the classification of individual pixels. In this context, classification means deciding to which classes the pixels in an image belong. It is a pixelwise operation that does not take the neighbors of a pixel into account and it is sometimes called a value-to-label operation, since it assigns a label to each pixel based on the pixel value. Pixel classification is often used as an initial step in image-based diagnostic systems.

An example can be seen in Fig. 9.1 where a computed tomography (CT) head image has been classified. The pixels have been classified as background (gray), bone (red), trabeculae[1] (green), or soft-tissue (blue). The result is a label image as described in Sect. 2.4.3.

In the following, these two questions will be answered:

1. Given a pixel value somewhere in an image, how do we assign a label to that pixel?
2. How do we decide how many classes and which classes it is possible for an image to contain?

Classification can be defined more formally as

Given a pixel value $v \in \mathbb{R}$, classify it as belonging to one of the k classes $C = c_1, \ldots, c_k$

In our example, there are $k = 4$ classes $C = \{c_1 = \text{background}, c_2 = \text{soft-tissue}, c_3 = \text{trabeculae}, c_4 = \text{bone}\}$. To perform the classification we need a *classification rule*:

$$c : \mathbb{R} \to \{c_1, \ldots, c_k\} \, ,$$

---

[1]Trabeculae is the spongy bone located inside the hard bone.

© Springer Nature Switzerland AG 2020
R. R. Paulsen and T. B. Moeslund, *Introduction to Medical Image Analysis*,
Undergraduate Topics in Computer Science,
https://doi.org/10.1007/978-3-030-39364-9_9

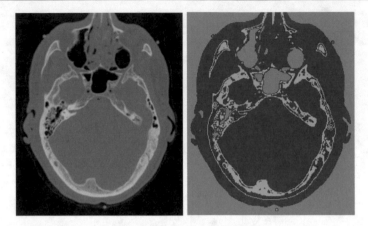

Fig. 9.1 Classification of a head CT image. To the left, the raw CT image. To the right the four classes identified in the image are shown with colors

that assigns pixels values to classes. The classification rule divides the possible pixel value range into limited intervals. The CT image in Fig. 9.1 is a gray-level image meaning that the value of a pixel is $v \in [0; 255]$.[2] By manual inspection we have found that the background pixel values typically are 4, soft-tissue pixels are 67, trabeculae pixels are 95, and bone pixels 150. A simple classification rule is therefore:

$$c(v) = \begin{cases} \text{background if } v \le (4+67)/2 \\ \text{soft-tissue} \quad \text{if } (4+67)/2 < v \le (67+95)/2 \\ \text{trabeculae} \quad \text{if } (67+95)/2 < v \le (95+150)/2 \\ \text{bone} \qquad \quad \text{if } v > (95+150)/2 \end{cases}$$

When a classification rule is determined, an entire image can be classified by applying the rule to all pixels in the image. As can be seen in Fig. 9.1, it works reasonably well on this image. However, many pixels are not correctly classified. In cases that are more difficult it is better to use more sophisticated training methods as will be described in the following sections.

9.1 Training

An important goal in many image analysis algorithms is to be able to *simulate* the performance of the best human experts. An example is to make an algorithm that can diagnose breast cancer as accurately as the best human experts can. A common approach is to *train* the algorithm by feeding it results produced by human experts.

---

[2]CT images are normally stored as 16-bit images. For this example, the image has been transformed into an 8-bit image.

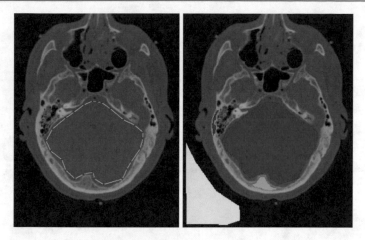

Fig. 9.2 Expert annotation of a head CT image. To the left is the selection tool used to mark a part of the soft-tissue. To the right the four regions are shown (red = bone, blue = soft-tissue, green = trabeculae, and yellow = background)

To continue with our example, a human expert has been asked to mark areas containing background, soft-tissue, trabeculae, and bone in a CT image using a simple drawing tool. This process is also called *annotation*. The expert's results can be seen in Fig. 9.2, where it should be noted that the expert has only pointed out representative regions and not every region containing for example bone. An important aspect is that training is only done once. However, it must be assumed that the images that should be classified are acquired using very similar capture conditions.[3] In the example, it is the expert that decides the number of possible classes, and that is often the case since it is closely correlated with the nature of the image. Alternatively, *unsupervised* methods exist. However, these are beyond the scope of this text.

So how do we learn from these annotations? An initial step is to inspect the histograms of the pixel values in the annotated regions. Secondly, some simple statistics for the pixel values in the regions can be computed. The histogram for the data in our head CT example can be seen in Fig. 9.3. The average pixel value μ and the standard deviation σ are also calculated for each class as seen in Table 9.1. By looking at the histogram it can be seen that the four classes are separated. However, it is also seen that there is an overlap between the soft-tissue and the trabeculae pixel values. Furthermore, the standard deviation of the trabeculae pixel values is larger than the others are. This is important since it tells something about the homogeneity of the tissue and will be examined later.

---

[3]The capture conditions are the parameters used when taken the picture.

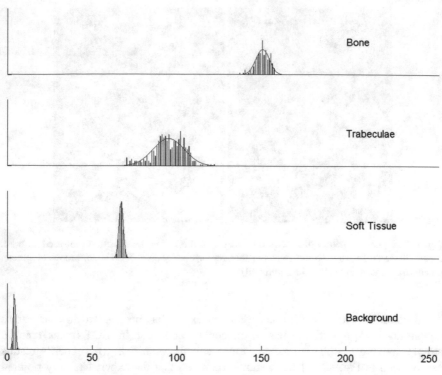

Fig. 9.3 Histograms of the pixel values in the annotated regions. The red line is a fitted Gaussian distribution

Table 9.1 Classwise pixel value statistics

Class (c_i)	Average pixel value (μ_i)	Standard deviation (σ_i)
Background	4.3	0.74
Soft-tissue	66.8	1.3
Trabeculae	95.9	9.3
Bone	150.2	3.95

9.2 Minimum Distance Classification

Based on the statistics of the gray levels in the training regions a simple classifier called the *minimum distance classifier* can be defined:

Given k classes and let μ_i be the average pixel values in the training set of class i. The minimum distance classifier assigns a pixel to the class i for whom the distance from the pixel value v to μ_i is minimum.

Table 9.2 Class ranges from the shortest distance classifier

Class	Pixel value range
Background	[0, 36]
Soft-tissue	[36, 81]
Trabeculae	[81, 123]
Bone	[123, 255]

In our case, the distance is calculated as the absolute difference between the pixel value and the class average:

$$d_i(v, \mu_i) = \|v - \mu_i\| . \tag{9.1}$$

The trained classes from the head CT example are used to classify the pixels in an image. For a pixel with value $v = 78$ the class distances are calculated: $d_{background} = 73.7$, $d_{Soft\text{-}tissue} = 11.2$, $d_{trabeculae} = 17.9$, and $d_{bone} = 72.2$. The pixel is therefore classified as soft-tissue. As can be seen, the minimum distance classifier divides the possible pixel values into ranges, that determine which class a given pixel values belongs to. The pixel value ranges from the example can be seen in Table 9.2. The ranges are calculated to have endpoints exactly where the distance between two neighboring classes is equal. For example $d_{Soft\text{-}tissue} = d_{trabeculae}$, when $v = (\mu_{Soft\text{-}tissue} + \mu_{trabeculae})/2$.

While the minimum distance classifier works well when the classes are well separated it is usually not the best choice if the classes are overlapping. A more sophisticated classifier that takes the shape of the histogram of each class into account is described next. In our example, and overlap between the trabeculae and soft-tissue classes exists and it could therefore be worth investigating more advanced methods.

9.3   Parametric Classification

In the minimum distance classifier, the only information that is used about the trained classes is the pixel value averages. When looking at the histograms in Fig. 9.3, it can be seen that it is not only the position of the average that makes the classes different. The classes also have different pixel value variance, which can also be seen in Table 9.1. This tells something about how well defined the class is. While the background has very little variance and is therefore very well defined, the trabeculae have a larger variance and this can lead to situations where it is uncertain if a pixel is really trabeculae.

To be able to use the extra information that is in the *shape* of the histogram, we need a way to describe this shape. A solution is to use a function that *looks like* the histogram to represent each class. This is also called a *parametric representation* of the histogram. In addition, it is also desirable to be able to describe as much information about the histogram with the fewest parameters as possible. A commonly used representation is the normal distribution that is also called the Gaussian distribution. The probability density function (PDF) is

$$f(x) = \frac{1}{\sigma\sqrt{2\pi}} \exp\left(-\frac{(x-\mu)^2}{2\sigma^2}\right) . \tag{9.2}$$

It can be seen that only two parameters, the mean value μ, and the variance σ^2 are needed to describe the Gaussian. Given a set of n values, $v_1, v_2, \ldots, v_n$, that are for example training pixel values, the parameters of the Gaussian distribution that fits these data can be estimated using

$$\hat{\mu} = \frac{1}{n}\sum_{i=1}^{n} v_i . \tag{9.3}$$

$$\hat{\sigma}^2 = \frac{1}{n-1}\sum_{i=1}^{n}(v_i - \hat{\mu})^2 , \tag{9.4}$$

where the "hat" over μ and σ means estimated values. The histogram of the annotated trabeculae pixel values can be seen in Fig. 9.4 together with the estimated Gaussian distribution. The plotted Gaussian is scaled (in height) to fit the plot of the histogram. It can be seen that the pixel values are not perfectly matching the Gaussian distribution. However, it is still a usable approximation.

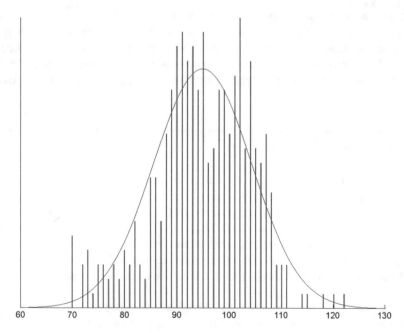

Fig. 9.4 The histogram of the annotated trabeculae pixel values together with the estimated Gaussian distribution. The plot of the Gaussian is scaled (in height) to fit the histogram

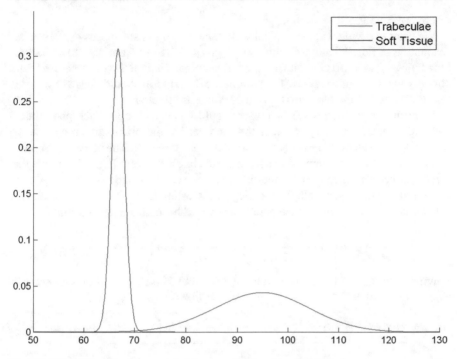

Fig. 9.5 Fitted Gaussians for annotated tissue and trabeculae pixel values

From the previous section, we learnt that the minimum distance classification is suited for classes that are well separated. Let us therefore examine two classes that are not so well separated. In Fig. 9.5, the fitted Gaussian distributions for the annotated trabeculae and soft-tissue pixel values are shown. The two classes seem to be well separated. Let us try to use the minimum distance classifier on a pixel with value $v = 78$. As demonstrated in an earlier example, this pixel will be classified as soft-tissue. If the learnt parametric representation of soft-tissue values are inspected (Fig. 9.5), it suddenly seems very unreasonable that this pixel should be soft-tissue. Instead, it should be classified as trabeculae. This change of decision is of course due to the variance of the two classes. A better choice of ranges should be based on the parametric description. One approach is to compare the parametric description for each class for a given pixel value and the class is selected as the one with the highest value of the parametric description. The parametric description of the pixel values of the soft-tissue is

$$f_1(v) = \frac{1}{\sigma_1 \sqrt{2\pi}} \exp\left(-\frac{(v - \mu_1)^2}{2\sigma_1^2}\right) , \tag{9.5}$$

where $\mu_1 = 66.8$ and $\sigma_1 = 1.3$. The parametric description for the trabeculae pixel values is

$$f_2(v) = \frac{1}{\sigma_2 \sqrt{2\pi}} \exp\left(-\frac{(v - \mu_2)^2}{2\sigma_2^2}\right) , \tag{9.6}$$

where $\mu_2 = 95.9$ and $\sigma_2 = 9.3$.

We want to decide whether a pixel with value $v = 78$ is soft-tissue or trabeculae. Evaluation of Eqs. 9.5 and 9.6 with $v = 78$ gives $f_1(78) \approx 0$ and $f_2(78) = 0.0083$. Since $f_2 > f_1$, the pixel is classified as trabeculae. This method can be used with not only two but many classes. The parametric description should then be evaluated for all classes and the one with the highest value is selected.

Using this method, several functions should be evaluated for each pixel that is classified. This is not very efficient. As seen earlier, the pixel value range can be subdivided into class ranges as seen in for example Table 9.2. The question is how to compute these ranges when using a parametric classifier. From Fig. 9.5 it seems that a good choice for the range delimiter is where the two distributions cross. However, finding that value is surprisingly complex. If the estimated Gaussian parameters for soft-tissue are μ_1 and σ_1 and the parameters for trabeculae are μ_2 and σ_2, then

$$\frac{1}{\sigma_1\sqrt{2\pi}} \exp\left(-\frac{(v - \mu_1)^2}{2\sigma_1^2}\right) = \frac{1}{\sigma_2\sqrt{2\pi}} \exp\left(-\frac{(v - \mu_2)^2}{2\sigma_2^2}\right)$$

Solving with respect to the pixel value v, turns out to be the solution of a second-degree polynomial. The two solutions are as follows:

$$\frac{\sigma_1^2\mu_2 - \sigma_2^2\mu_1 \pm \sqrt{-\sigma_1^2\sigma_2^2\left(2\mu_2\mu_1 - \mu_2^2 - 2\sigma_2^2\ln\left(\frac{\sigma_2}{\sigma_1}\right) - \mu_1^2 + 2\sigma_1^2\ln\left(\frac{\sigma_2}{\sigma_1}\right)\right)}}{-\sigma_2^2 + \sigma_1^2}$$

The range delimiter is chosen to be the solution that is closest to the range delimiter found by the minimum distance approach. Using the above formula it is found that the Gaussian for the soft-tissue and for the trabeculae cross at $v = 71$. The complete pixel value class range computed with the parametric classifier can be seen in Table 9.3. The greatest change when comparing to Table 9.2 is that the range of trabeculae pixels is significantly extended. The result of using the parametric classifier on the head CT image can be seen in Fig. 9.6. Compared to the classification seen in Fig. 9.1, the trabeculae is much more prominent. From an anatomical viewpoint it seems that some cortical bone is misclassified as trabeculae.

A common approach is to pre-compute a look-up-table that maps given pixel values to classes. This is only done once and therefore it is feasible to compare the parametric description of all the classes when computing the look-up-table.

Table 9.3 Class ranges from the parametric classifier

Class	Pixel value range
Background	[0, 27]
Soft-tissue	[27, 71]
Trabeculae	[71, 133]
Bone	[133, 255]

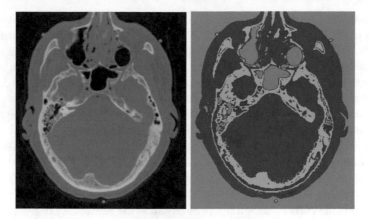

Fig. 9.6 Classification of a head CT image. To the left, the raw CT image. To the right the four classes identified in the image are shown with colors

9.4 Bayesian Classification

In the previous sections, it was assumed that a standard image contains approximately the same amount of pixels from all the classes. The classification of the pixels is therefore done by comparing the *normalized* parametric descriptions. Normalized means that the area under the curve is equal to one. In some cases, some classes are much more present in the image than other classes and in this case the normalized representation is not ideal. For example, it is easy to see on the CT scan of the head (Fig. 9.6 left) that there are more background pixels and soft-tissue pixels than trabeculae and bone pixels.

Suppose that a trained radiologist tells that a normal CT scan contains approximately 40% background, 30% soft-tissue, 20% bone, and 10% trabeculae. This means that if a pixel is selected at random its probability of being soft-tissue is 30%. These estimated percentages give the probability of a pixel belonging to a class even before looking at its value [6]. This is called the *a prior probabilities*.[4] This suggests that we should use this to weight the decisions made using the parametric classification. Bayesian classification provides a framework for doing exactly that.

Bayesian Classification or more formally Bayesian Maximum Likelihood Classification is an important method from statistical decision theory. It is based on Bayes formula:

$$P(c_i|v) = \frac{P(v|c_i)P(c_i)}{P(v)} \ . \tag{9.7}$$

This formula is not easy to understand or apply at first. In the following, we will describe both why it is useful and how to practically use it. The formula allows us

---

[4]The word *prior* means *before*. *Prior knowledge* means therefore *something that is known before*.

to compute the *posterior probability* $P(c_i|v)$. That is the probability of a given pixel belongs to the class c_i when the value of the pixel is v. Exactly like the parametric classifier, the class is chosen to be the one with the highest posterior probability.

As an example, let us assume that we know how to use Bayes formula and that we want to classify a pixel with value $v = 75$. Using the Bayes formula, we compute the posterior probability for our four classes: $c_1 =$ background, $c_2 =$ soft-tissue, $c_3 =$ trabeculae, and $c_4 =$ bone. The posterior probability turns out to be highest for $c_3 =$ trabeculae and we therefore set pixel label to trabeculae.

In Bayes formula, $P(c_i)$ is the *prior probability*. In our case, it is the probability that a chosen pixel belongs to a given class, without looking at its pixel value. Using the radiologists advise we have $P(\text{background}) = 40\%$, $P(\text{bone}) = 20\%$, $P(\text{trabeculae}) = 10\%$, and $P(\text{soft-tissue}) = 30\%$.

$P(v|c_i)$ is the *class conditional probability*. It is the probability of a pixel having the value v when the pixel belongs to class c_i. The parametric descriptions of the class histograms seen in Fig. 9.3 give an approximation of the *class conditional probability*. It can be seen that it is very unlikely that a pixel with value $v = 100$ is a background, soft-tissue, or bone pixel. However, there is a high probability that it is a trabeculae pixel. $P(v|c_i)$ can therefore be described using the parametric description of the class histogram. Finally, $P(v)$ acts as a normalizing constant and is ignored (set to one) in the following.

The steps needed to construct and use a Bayesian classifier are as follows:

1. Identify the number of classes using common sense and expert inputs.
2. Mark the chosen classes as areas in a training image. It is not necessary that all pixels in the training image are marked.
3. Compute parametric description of each class histogram. This is the estimate of $P(v|c_i)$.
4. Estimate the prior probabilities $P(c_i)$ using either expert input or by inspecting the training image.
5. Classify each pixel in the image by computing $P(c_i|v)$ for each class and select the class with the highest probability. In practise,

$$P(c_i|v) = P(v|c_i)P(c_i) \, , \tag{9.8}$$

since we ignore $P(v)$.

Using the Gaussian parametric description, $P(c_i|v)$ is computed as

$$P(c_i|v) = P(c_i)\frac{1}{\sqrt{2\pi}\sigma_i} \exp\left(-\frac{(v-\mu_i)^2}{2\sigma_i^2}\right) \, , \tag{9.9}$$

where μ_i and σ_i are the pixel value average and standard deviation of class c_i. From the previous sections, we have that the parametric description of the pixel values of the soft-tissue is

$$f_1(v) = \frac{1}{\sigma_1\sqrt{2\pi}} \exp\left(-\frac{(v-\mu_1)^2}{2\sigma_1^2}\right) \, , \tag{9.10}$$

where $\mu_1 = 66.8$ and $\sigma_1 = 1.3$. The parametric description for the trabeculae pixel values is therefore

$$f_2(v) = \frac{1}{\sigma_2\sqrt{2\pi}} \exp\left(-\frac{(v-\mu_2)^2}{2\sigma_2^2}\right) , \qquad (9.11)$$

where $\mu_2 = 95.9$ and $\sigma_2 = 9.3$. We want to decide whether a pixel with value $v = 78$ is soft-tissue or trabeculae. Evaluation of Eqs. 9.10 and 9.11 with $v = 78$ gives $f_1(78) = 0$ and $f_2(78) = 0.0083$. These two values are now multiplied with the prior probability for soft-tissue (30%) and trabeculae (10%) to create the posterior probabilities:

$$P(\text{soft-tissue}|v = 78) = 0.3 \cdot f_1(78) = 0$$

and

$$P(\text{trabeculae}|v = 78) = 0.1 \cdot f_2(78) = 0.00083$$

Since $P(\text{trabeculae}|v = 78) > P(\text{soft-tissue}|v = 78)$, the pixel is classified as trabeculae. The exponential in Eq. 9.9 can be avoided by taking the logarithm. If the constant term is dropped, the equation can be written as

$$\ln(P(c_i|v) = \ln P(c_i) - \ln \sigma_i - \frac{(v-\mu_i)^2}{2\sigma_i^2}. \qquad (9.12)$$

Since $P(c_i)$ and $\ln \sigma_i$ can be pre-computed, the estimation of the maximum a posterior estimate can be made faster using this method.

9.5   When to Use the Different Classifiers

It is very difficult to choose the correct classification strategy without looking at some example data and there is seldom one correct approach. Some general advices can be given though. If your data consists of well-separated classes with little pixel value variation within the classes, the minimum distance classifier is a good choice. If you have different variations within the classes and there are overlap between the classes, a good choice is the parametric classifier. If on top of that, some classes are much more present in the training set (a lot of soft-tissue and very little bone for example); the Bayesian classifier should be considered.

Geometric Transformations

10

Most people have tried to do a geometric transformation of an image when preparing a presentation or when manipulating an image. The two most well-known are perhaps rotation and scaling, but others exist. In this chapter, we will describe how such transformations operate and discuss the issues that need to be considered when doing such transformations.

The term "geometric" transformation refers to the class of image transformation where the geometry of the image is changed but the actual pixel values remain unchanged.[1]

Let us recall from the previous chapters that an image is defined as $f(x, y)$, where $f(\cdot)$ denotes the intensity or gray-level value and (x, y) defines the position of the pixel. After a geometric transformation the image is transformed into a new image denoted $g(x', y')$, where the tic (') means position in $g(x, y)$. This might seem confusing, but we need some way of stating the position before the transformation (x, y) and after the transformation (x', y').

As mentioned above the actual intensity values are not changed by the geometric transformation, but the positions of the pixels are (from (x, y) to (x', y')). So if $f(2, 3) = 120$ then in general $g(2, 3) \neq 120$. A geometric transformation basically calculates where the pixel at position (x, y) in $f(x, y)$ will be located in $g(x', y')$. That is, a mapping from (x, y) to (x', y'). We denote this mapping as

$$x' = A_x(x, y) \tag{10.1}$$

$$y' = A_y(x, y), \tag{10.2}$$

where $A_x(x, y)$ and $A_y(x, y)$ are both functions, which map from the position (x, y) to x' and y', respectively.

---

[1]For readers interested in a quick refreshment or introduction to linear algebra—in particular vectors and matrices—please refer to Appendix B.

© Springer Nature Switzerland AG 2020

R. R. Paulsen and T. B. Moeslund, *Introduction to Medical Image Analysis*,
Undergraduate Topics in Computer Science,
https://doi.org/10.1007/978-3-030-39364-9_10

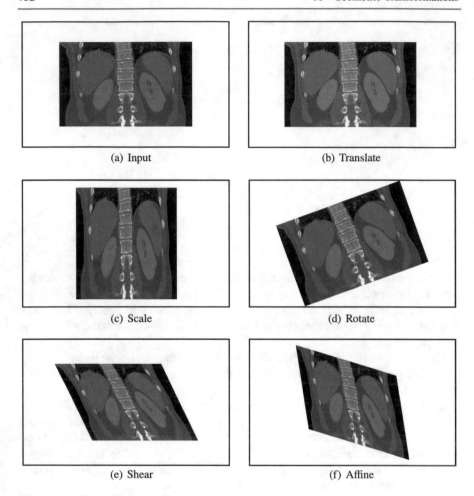

Fig. 10.1   Different affine transformations

10.1   Affine Transformations

The class of *affine transformations* covers four different transformations, which are illustrated in Fig. 10.1. These are: translation, rotation, scaling, and shearing.

10.1.1   Translation

Let us now look at the transformations in Fig. 10.1 and define their concrete mapping equations. Translation is simply a matter of shifting the image horizontally and vertically with a given offset (measured in pixels) denoted Δx and Δy. For translation the mapping is thus defined as

$$x' = x + \Delta x \atop y' = y + \Delta y \Rightarrow \begin{bmatrix} x' \\ y' \end{bmatrix} = \begin{bmatrix} x \\ y \end{bmatrix} + \begin{bmatrix} \Delta x \\ \Delta y \end{bmatrix} \tag{10.3}$$

So if $\Delta x = 100$ and $\Delta y = 100$, then each pixel is shifted 100 pixels in both the x- and y-direction.

10.1.2 Scaling

When scaling an image, it is made smaller or bigger in the x- and/or y-direction. Say we have an image of size 300×200 and we wish to transform it into a 600×100 image. The x-direction is then scaled by: $600/300 = 2$. We denote this the x-scale factor and write it as $S_x = 2$. Similarly $S_y = 100/200 = 1/2$. Together this means that the pixel in the image $f(x, y)$ at position $(x, y) = (100, 100)$ is mapped to a new position in the image $g(x', y')$, namely, $(x', y') = (100 \cdot 2, 100 \cdot 1/2) = (200, 50)$. In general, scaling is expressed as follows:

$$x' = x \cdot S_x \atop y' = y \cdot S_y \Rightarrow \begin{bmatrix} x' \\ y' \end{bmatrix} = \begin{bmatrix} S_x & 0 \\ 0 & S_y \end{bmatrix} \cdot \begin{bmatrix} x \\ y \end{bmatrix} \tag{10.4}$$

10.1.3 Rotation

When rotating an image, as illustrated in Fig. 10.1d, we need to define the amount of rotation in terms of an angle. We denote this angle θ meaning that each pixel in $f(x, y)$ is rotated θ degrees. The transformation is defined as

$$x' = x \cdot \cos\theta - y \cdot \sin\theta \atop y' = x \cdot \sin\theta + y \cdot \cos\theta \Rightarrow \begin{bmatrix} x' \\ y' \end{bmatrix} = \begin{bmatrix} \cos\theta & -\sin\theta \\ \sin\theta & \cos\theta \end{bmatrix} \cdot \begin{bmatrix} x \\ y \end{bmatrix} \tag{10.5}$$

Note that the rotation is done counterclockwise. If we wish to do a clockwise rotation we can either use $-\theta$ or change the transformation to

$$x' = x \cdot \cos\theta + y \cdot \sin\theta \atop y' = -x \cdot \sin\theta + y \cdot \cos\theta \Rightarrow \begin{bmatrix} x' \\ y' \end{bmatrix} = \begin{bmatrix} \cos\theta & \sin\theta \\ -\sin\theta & \cos\theta \end{bmatrix} \cdot \begin{bmatrix} x \\ y \end{bmatrix} \tag{10.6}$$

10.1.4 Shearing

To shear an image means to shift pixels either horizontally, B_x, or vertically, B_y. The difference from translation is that the shifting is not done by the same amount, but depends on where in the image a pixel is. In Fig. 10.1e $B_x = 0$ and $B_y = -0.5$. The transformation is defined as

$$x' = x + y \cdot B_x \atop y' = x \cdot B_y + y \Rightarrow \begin{bmatrix} x' \\ y' \end{bmatrix} = \begin{bmatrix} 1 & B_x \\ B_y & 1 \end{bmatrix} \cdot \begin{bmatrix} x \\ y \end{bmatrix} \tag{10.7}$$

10.1.5 Combining the Transformations

The four transformations can be combined in all kinds of different ways by multiplying the matrices in different orders, yielding a number of different transformations. One is shown in Fig. 10.1f. Instead of defining the scale factors, the shearing factors and the rotation angle, it is common to merge these three transformations to one matrix. The combination of the four transformations is therefore defined as

$$
\begin{aligned}
x' &= a_1 \cdot x + a_2 \cdot y + a_3 \\
y' &= b_1 \cdot x + b_2 \cdot y + b_3
\end{aligned}
\Rightarrow
\begin{bmatrix} x' \\ y' \end{bmatrix}
=
\begin{bmatrix} a_1 & a_2 \\ b_1 & b_2 \end{bmatrix}
\cdot
\begin{bmatrix} x \\ y \end{bmatrix}
+
\begin{bmatrix} a_3 \\ b_3 \end{bmatrix},
\tag{10.8}
$$

and this is the affine transformation. Below the relationships between Eq. 10.8 and the four above mentioned transformations are listed. Often *homogeneous coordinates*

	a_1	a_2	a_3	b_1	b_2	b_3
Translation	1	0	Δ_x	0	1	Δ_y
Scaling	S_x	0	0	0	S_y	0
Rotation	$\cos\theta$	$-\sin\theta$	0	$\sin\theta$	$\cos\theta$	0
Shearing	1	B_x	0	B_y	1	0

are used when implementing the transformation since they make further calculations faster. In homogeneous coordinates, the affine transformation becomes

$$
\begin{bmatrix} x' \\ y' \\ 1 \end{bmatrix}
=
\begin{bmatrix} a_1 & a_2 & a_3 \\ b_1 & b_2 & b_3 \\ 0 & 0 & 1 \end{bmatrix}
\cdot
\begin{bmatrix} x \\ y \\ 1 \end{bmatrix},
\tag{10.9}
$$

where $a_3 = \Delta x$ and $b_3 = \Delta y$.

10.2 Backward Mapping

In terms of programming, the affine transformation consists of two steps. First the coefficients of the affine transformation matrix are defined. Second we go though all pixels in the image $f(x, y)$ one at a time (using two for-loops) and find the position of each pixel in $g(x', y')$ using Eq. 10.9. This process is known as *forward mapping*, i.e., mapping each pixel from $f(x, y)$ to $g(x', y')$.

At a first glance this simple process seems to be fine, but unfortunately it is not. Let us have a closer look at the scaling transformation in order to understand the nature of the problem. Say we have an image of size 300×200 and want to scale this to 510×200. From above we can calculate that $S_x = 510/300 = 1.7$ and $S_y = 200/200 = 1$. Using Eq. 10.4 the pixel positions in a row of $f(x, y)$ are mapped in the following manner:

We can observe that "holes" are present in $g(x', y')$. If for example 10.2 is rounded off to 10 and 11.9–12, then $x' = 11$ will have no value, hence a hole in the image output. If the scaling factor is smaller than 1 then a related problem would occur, namely,

x	0	1	2	3	4	5	6	7	8	$\cdots$	300
x'	0	1.7	3.4	5.1	6.8	8.5	10.2	11.9	13.6	$\cdots$	510

that multiple pixels from $f(x, y)$ are mapped to the same pixel in $g(x', y')$. Similar problems are evident for shearing and rotation. In Fig. 10.2 the forward mapping is illustrated.

The solution is to avoid forward mapping and instead use *backward mapping*. Backward mapping maps from $g(x', y')$ to $f(x, y)$. That is, it goes through the *output image*, $g(x', y')$, one pixel at a time (using two for-loops) and for each position (x', y') it uses the *inverse transformation* to calculate (x, y). That is, it finds out where in the input image a pixel must come from in order to be mapped to (x', y'). The principle is illustrated in Fig. 10.2. The inverse transformation is found by matrix inversion of the transformation matrix as

$$\begin{bmatrix} x \\ y \\ 1 \end{bmatrix} = \begin{bmatrix} a_1 & a_2 & a_3 \\ b_1 & b_2 & b_3 \\ 0 & 0 & 1 \end{bmatrix}^{-1} \cdot \begin{bmatrix} x' \\ y' \\ 1 \end{bmatrix} \qquad (10.10)$$

For scaling, rotation, and shearing the inverse matrices look like the following:

$$\text{Scaling: } \begin{bmatrix} 1/S_x & 0 \\ 0 & 1/S_y \end{bmatrix} \text{Rotation: } \begin{bmatrix} \cos\theta & \sin\theta \\ -\sin\theta & \cos\theta \end{bmatrix} \qquad (10.11)$$

$$\text{Shearing: } \frac{1}{1 - B_x B_y} \begin{bmatrix} 1 & -B_x \\ -B_y & 1 \end{bmatrix} \qquad (10.12)$$

As can be seen in Fig. 10.2 backward mapping is very likely to result in a value of (x, y) which is not possible. For example, what is the intensity value of $f(3.4, 7.9)$? It is undefined and we therefore *interpolate* in order to find an appropriate intensity

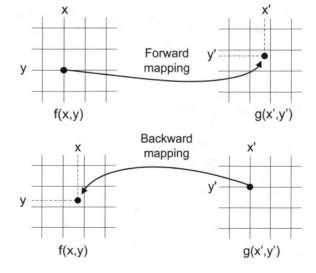

Fig. 10.2 Forward and backward mapping

Fig. 10.3 Bilinear
interpolation. The final pixel
value becomes a weighted
sum of the four nearest pixel
values

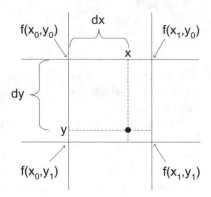

value. The most simple form of interpolation is called zero-order interpolation. It rounds off to the value of the nearest possible pixel, i.e., $f(3.4, 7.9) \rightarrow f(3, 8)$. A better, but also more computational demanding, approach is to apply first-order interpolation (aka bilinear interpolation), which weights the intensity values of the four nearest pixels according to how close they are. The principle is illustrated in Fig. 10.3. The area of the square wherein (x, y) is located is 1. Now imagine that we use the position (x, y) to divide this square into four subregions. The area of each of these subregions defines the weight of one of the four nearest pixels. That is, the area $dx \cdot dy$ becomes the weight for the pixel $f(x_1, y_1)$ and so forth. The final intensity value is then found as

$$
\begin{aligned}
g(x', y') = & f(x_0, y_0) \cdot (1 - dx)(1 - dy) \\
& + f(x_1, y_0) \cdot (dx)(1 - dy) \\
& + f(x_0, y_1) \cdot (1 - dx)(dy) \\
& + f(x_1, y_1) \cdot (dx \cdot dy).
\end{aligned}
\tag{10.13}
$$

Note that this equation can be rewritten more compactly for an efficient software implementation. Note also that more advanced methods for interpolation exist, but this is beyond the scope of this text.

10.3   Profile Analysis

Sometimes it can be useful to get an idea of the gray levels around important features in the image. A gray-level profile is a powerful tool for that. A gray level profile maps the gray values as a function of traveled distance when traveling from one point in the image to another. In Fig. 10.4 an X-ray image of a hand is seen. A profile has been selected going from the upper right corner and down. To the left, the gray levels on the profile are plotted as function of traveled distance. The five metacarpal bones are clearly seen as double peaks in the profile. Each bone creates a double peak because it is hollow.

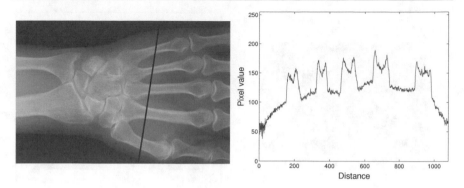

Fig. 10.4 Profile analysis on an X-ray image of a hand. The profile goes from top to bottom

To compute a profile, the user starts by placing a start point p_s and an end point p_e in the image. We now need to find the points on the line from p_s to p_e and sample the gray level in these points. This is done by first finding the length of the line:

$$l = \| p_e - p_s \|,\tag{10.14}$$

where we use the vector length as described in Sect. B.5 in Appendix B. The next step is to compute the unit vector based on profile line (see Eq. B.15 in Sect. B.5):

$$\vec{u} = \frac{p_e - p_s}{l},\tag{10.15}$$

The points on the profile can now be computed as

$$p = p_s + i \cdot \vec{u},\tag{10.16}$$

where $i = 0, 1, \ldots, l_r - 1, l_r$. Here l_r is the rounded version of l. Since the points p are not necessarily placed directly in the middle of the pixels, bilinear interpolation is used to sample the pixel values.

10.4 Other Geometric Transformations

There exist a number of other geometric transformations. Some are used for correcting errors in images while others are used for generating "errors" in images. The latter type of transformations can be compared to the magic mirrors found in entertainment parks, where, e.g., the head of the person facing the mirror is enlarged in a strange way while the legs are made smaller. Such transformations are said to be *non-linear* as opposed to the affine transformation which is linear. What is meant by this is that transformations which can be written as a product between a vector and some matrix (for example, as in Eq. 10.9) are said to be linear. Transformations involving, for example, trigonometric operations, square roots, etc. are said to be non-linear. Examples of non-linear transformations are illustrated in Fig. 10.5.

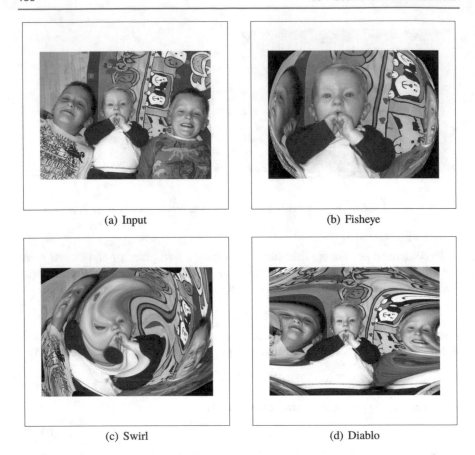

(a) Input   (b) Fisheye

(c) Swirl   (d) Diablo

Fig. 10.5 Different non-linear transformations

The actual process of transformation is similar to the one described above for the affine transformation except that more complicated (non-linear) math is applied, for example:

$$x' = a_1 \cdot x^2 + a_2 \cdot y^2 + a_3 \cdot xy + a_4 \cdot x + a_5 \cdot y + a_6 \qquad (10.17)$$

$$y' = b_1 \cdot x^2 + b_2 \cdot y^2 + b_3 \cdot xy + b_4 \cdot x + b_5 \cdot y + b_6. \qquad (10.18)$$

An alternative to *one* complicated transformation for the entire image is to apply a number of simpler transformations locally. Using the analogy to magic mirrors, this corresponds to the glass of the mirror being shaped differently depending on its position on the mirror. Often such transformations are denoted *warpings*. Figure 10.6 shows an example of how the input image is divided into triangles, which are then each mapped by a simple (affine) transform.

Another use of warping is found in *morphing*. Morphing is the process of mapping one image into another image. This is seen in, for example, in TV commercials where a wild animal is mapped into a beautiful woman. Morphing is based on knowing

Fig. 10.6 An example of warping, where a 4×4 image is divided into 32 triangles each having its own affine transformation

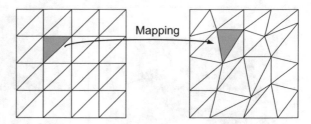

where a number of keypoints in one image should end up in the other image, e.g., the position of eyes, ears, and mouth. These points are used to calculate appropriate coefficients for the warping. Besides changing the shape of the image using warping, morphing also interpolates the intensities of the two images using alpha blending, see Sect. 4.5.1.

10.5 Homography

As mentioned above a geometric transformation can also be used to correct errors in an image. Imagine a telescope capturing an image of a star constellation. The image is likely to be distorted by the fact that light is bent in space due to the gravitational forces of the stars and also by the changing conditions in the Earth's atmosphere. Since the nature of these phenomena is known, the transformation they enforced on the image can be compensated for by applying the inverse transformation.

Another, and perhaps more relevant, error that can be corrected by a geometric transformation is *keystoning*. A keystone is the top-most block in an arch, i.e., an arch-shaped doorway. Since the keystone is wedge-shaped it is used to describe wedge-shaped images. Such an image is obtained when capturing a square using a tilted camera or when projecting an image onto a tilted plane, see Fig. 10.7. Since this is a common phenomenon most projectors have a built-in function, which can correct for keystoning.

Let us investigate the correction of keystoning in more depth by looking at a concrete example. Imagine you are designing a simple game where a projector projects circles onto a table and a camera captures your finger when touching the table. The purpose of the game could then be to see how many circles you can touch in a predefined time period. For such a system to work you need, among other things, to know what a detected pixel coordinate (the position of the finger) corresponds to in the image projected onto the table. If both camera and projector are tilted with respect to the table, then two keystone errors are actually present. In general, the geometric transformation which maps from one plane (camera image) to another (projected image) is known as a projective *transformation* or *homography*. It can be calculated in the following way using the *Direct Linear Transform* [3].

First have a look at Fig. 10.8 to see what we are dealing with. To the left you see an illustration of two coordinate systems. The (x, y) coordinate system is the

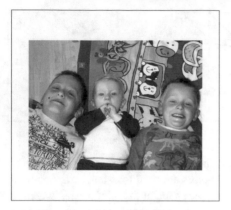 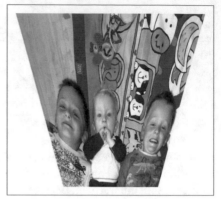

Fig. 10.7 Keystoning with the input image to the left and the keystoned image to the right

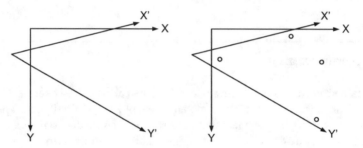

Fig. 10.8 The coordinate system of the image (x, y) and the coordinate system of the projector (x', y') seen from the image's point of view. Right: The circles are projected from the projector in order to find corresponding points in the two coordinate systems

coordinate system of the image and the (x', y') coordinate system is the coordinate system of the projector seen from the image's point of view. Or in other words, if you make the projector project two perpendicular arrows onto a plane (for example, a table) and capture a picture of the table, then the perpendicular arrows will look like the x' and y' arrows. So the transformation we are after should map from (x, y) to (x', y').

From the theory of Homography, we know that the mapping between the two coordinate systems is

$$
\begin{bmatrix} h \cdot x' \\ h \cdot y' \\ h \end{bmatrix} = \begin{bmatrix} a_1 \ a_2 \ a_3 \\ b_1 \ b_2 \ b_3 \\ c_1 \ c_2 \ 1 \end{bmatrix} \cdot \begin{bmatrix} x \\ y \\ 1 \end{bmatrix}. \tag{10.19}
$$

From this it follows that

$$
\frac{h \cdot x'}{h} = x' \qquad\qquad = \frac{a_1 \cdot x + a_2 \cdot y + a_3}{c_1 \cdot x + c_2 \cdot y + 1} \tag{10.20}
$$

$$
\frac{h \cdot y'}{h} = y' \qquad\qquad = \frac{b_1 \cdot x + b_2 \cdot y + b_3}{c_1 \cdot x + c_2 \cdot y + 1}. \tag{10.21}
$$

Rewriting into matrix form we have

$$\begin{bmatrix} x' \\ y' \end{bmatrix} = \begin{bmatrix} x & y & 1 & 0 & 0 & 0 & -x \cdot x' & -y \cdot x' \\ 0 & 0 & 0 & x & y & 1 & -x \cdot y' & -y \cdot y' \end{bmatrix} \cdot \mathbf{d}, \qquad (10.22)$$

where $\mathbf{d} = [a_1, a_2, a_3, b_1, b_2, b_3, c_1, c_2,]^T$.

In order to find the values of the coefficients we need to know the positions of four points in both coordinate systems, i.e., eight equations with eight unknowns. We could, for example, send out four points from the projector and then find their positions (automatic or manual) in the image, see Fig. 10.8B. Then we would have the positions of four corresponding points in both coordinate systems[2]:

$$(x_1, y_1) \leftrightarrow (x_1', y_1') \quad (x_2, y_2) \leftrightarrow (x_2', y_2') \quad (x_3, y_3) \leftrightarrow (x_3', y_3') \quad (x_4, y_4) \leftrightarrow (x_4', y_4').$$

If we enter these points into the equations we end up with the following linear system $\mathbf{e} = \mathbf{Kd}$:

$$\begin{bmatrix} x_1' \\ y_1' \\ x_2' \\ y_2' \\ x_3' \\ y_3' \\ x_4' \\ y_4' \end{bmatrix} = \begin{bmatrix} x_1 & y_1 & 1 & 0 & 0 & 0 & -x_1 \cdot x_1' & -y_1 \cdot x_1' \\ 0 & 0 & 0 & x_1 & y_1 & 1 & -x_1 \cdot y_1' & -y_1 \cdot y_1' \\ x_2 & y_2 & 1 & 0 & 0 & 0 & -x_2 \cdot x_2' & -y_2 \cdot x_2' \\ 0 & 0 & 0 & x_2 & y_2 & 1 & -x_2 \cdot y_2' & -y_2 \cdot y_2' \\ x_3 & y_3 & 1 & 0 & 0 & 0 & -x_3 \cdot x_3' & -y_3 \cdot x_3' \\ 0 & 0 & 0 & x_3 & y_3 & 1 & -x_3 \cdot y_3' & -y_3 \cdot y_3' \\ x_4 & y_4 & 1 & 0 & 0 & 0 & -x_4 \cdot x_4' & -y_4 \cdot x_4' \\ 0 & 0 & 0 & x_4 & y_4 & 1 & -x_4 \cdot y_4' & -y_4 \cdot y_4' \end{bmatrix} \cdot \begin{bmatrix} a_1 \\ a_2 \\ a_3 \\ b_1 \\ b_2 \\ b_3 \\ c_1 \\ c_2 \end{bmatrix}. \qquad (10.23)$$

The coefficients of the transformation are now found as $\mathbf{d} = \mathbf{K}^{-1}\mathbf{e}$, which is solved using linear algebra, see Appendix B.

It should be noted that the process of finding the transformation is often referred to as (camera) *calibration*.

---

[2]It is important that the four points you project, (x', y'), are spread out across the entire image. This will ensure a good transformation. If your points are too close together, then the transformation might not be applicable for the entire image, but only for the region wherein the points are located.

Image Registration

11

Imagine that two images have been taken of the same patient. The first image was taken before an operation and the second after the operation. It could be interesting if the two images could be used to determine what impact the operation had. The operation could, for example, involve the removal of a cancer in the liver and the images could help to determine if the cancer was completely removed. An obvious solution is to subtract the two images and examine the resulting difference image. However, the difference image will also be influenced by the fact that it is not physically possible to place a patient in exactly the same position during two scans. The way to deal with this problem is called *image registration*. Using image registration, two images can be aligned so they fit together in the best possible way. The subtraction and comparison of the images can then be done after the image registration. Formally, image registration is the process of determining a geometrical transformation (see Chap. 10) that aligns an image to another reference image. In other words, one image is moved, rotated, and perhaps stretched until it fits another image.

In medical image analysis, image registration is used, for example, to compute the changes in an individual patient over time (change monitoring) or to compare one patient with other patients. It is also very useful when combining images from different types of medical scanners or cameras (data fusion). In Fig. 11.1 corresponding slices of the same brain imaged with a magnetic resonance (MR) scanner and a computed tomography (CT) scanner, respectively, are shown. The two scanners have different spatial resolution, and the images have slightly different positions with respect to the anatomy due to different patient positioning in the scanners. If we want to consider the information in the images simultaneously, we must provide a geometrical transformation between the two images. For cancer diagnostics, a combination of CT and positron emission tomography (PET) imagery is often used—the CT images provide the anatomical information and the PET images the functional information. In practice, a combined PET-CT image is created by aligning the two images together and fusing the information in the images.

In image-guided intervention and minimally invasive surgery, optical images of surface structures and ultrasound images acquired inter-operatively must be regis-

© Springer Nature Switzerland AG 2020

R. R. Paulsen and T. B. Moeslund, *Introduction to Medical Image Analysis*,
Undergraduate Topics in Computer Science,
https://doi.org/10.1007/978-3-030-39364-9_11

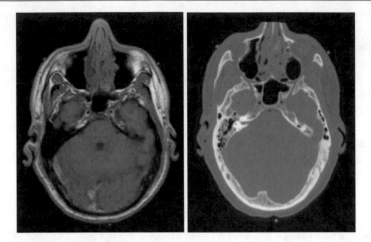

Fig. 11.1 Illustration of an MR-image and a CT image of the *same* brain. Notice how the MR-image is of different size and resolution

tered to preoperatively acquired MR and CT images providing the surgeon with an overview of detailed 3D anatomical structure during the operation.

Image registration is also very important when evaluating the progression of a disease or the effect of a treatment from images acquired at different time points, e.g., days, weeks, and years apart.

Sometimes the second image may be a computer-based anatomical "atlas", e.g., in the form of a generic image of a particular anatomy segmented and labeled which allows for automated image interpretation by transferred image labels to the image under study.

Finally, for population studies it is often of interest to compare images of many individuals, in order to quantify the biological variability. For example, is the hearing aid industry very interested in the variation of the shape of the human ear. By knowing, for example, the shape of the average ear and the major variation of this shape, better hearing aids can be designed that fit better to a larger group of people.

In image registration an image can both be a two-dimensional image, a three-dimensional array or for example a 3D surface. In the following, we will only consider standard two-dimensional images.

11.1   Feature-Based Image Registration

We will start by looking at image registration that is based on the idea of matching image features. An image feature can be a point or a line that is easy to recognize in all images. If we try to register two images of the human face, typical features would be the tip of the nose, the corners of the mouth, and the corners of the eyes.

To simplify this introduction we will narrow the topic further down to the so-called landmark-based image registration.

In landmark-based image registration, a set of corresponding landmarks is manually or semi-automatically placed in both images. Correspondence means that the landmarks must be placed on corresponding places in the two images. If, for example, landmark number 21 is placed on the tip of the nose in the first image, landmark number 21 should also be placed on the tip of the nose in the second image. Obviously, landmarks can only be placed on structures that are visible in both images. A landmark is sometimes called a *fiducial marker*. In the literature, landmarks have been known by various synonyms and been partitioned into various types. We will consider the three types defined by [2] in relation to biological shapes:

Anatomical landmark | a mark assigned by an expert that corresponds between objects in a biologically meaningful way.
Mathematical landmark | a mark that is located on a curve according to some mathematical or geometrical property (e.g., a point of maximum curvature).
Pseudo landmark | a mark that is constructed on a curve based on anatomical or mathematical landmarks (e.g. sampled equidistantly along an outline).

In Fig. 11.2 both anatomical, mathematical, and pseudo landmarks are shown on a hand. It is not always easy to place landmarks. In particular, it is very difficult to place consistent landmarks in 3D images and therefore it is a focus of recent research to automate this process or completely avoid it.

Assume that an expert has put landmarks on a pair of images. We call the image that is fixed for the *reference image* $\mathcal{R}$ and the image that is to be changed for the *template image* $\mathcal{T}$. The set of N landmarks placed in the reference image is

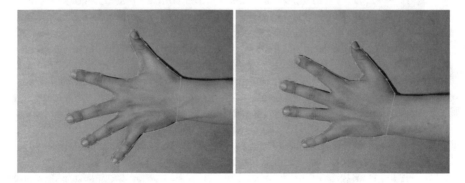

Fig. 11.2 Two images of the same hand. Each hand is annotated with 56 landmarks. Some landmarks are anatomical landmarks placed at the finger joints, others are mathematical landmarks placed at points of maximum surface curvatures, and a few of the landmarks are pseudo landmarks placed by sampling part of the curves equidistantly

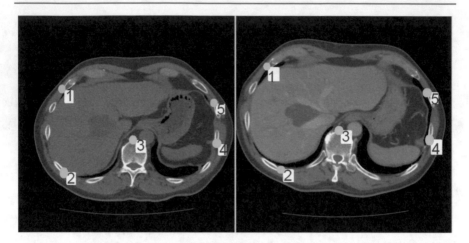

Fig. 11.3 A preoperative CT scan (the reference) is seen to the left and a postoperative CT scan (the template) is seen to the right. Five corresponding landmarks have been manually selected

Table 11.1 Manually selected landmarks in the reference image and in the template image from Fig. 11.3

i	a_i	b_i
1	(106.75, 178.75)	(74.125, 125.125)
2	(110.25, 374.25)	(108.875, 366.875)
3	(273.75, 299.75)	(246.125, 275.125)
4	(469.25, 306.75)	(459.125, 297.625)
5	(465.75, 212.75)	(456.625, 182.875)

$a_i \in \mathbb{R}^2, i = 1, \ldots, N$ and the set of N landmarks in the template image is $b_i \in \mathbb{R}^2$, $i = 1, \ldots, N$. Note that a_i and b_i are points and not scalar values. In the following, the landmarks are treated as vectors (as described in Sect. B.5).

As an example, a CT scan of a patient before surgery is seen (to the left) together with a CT scan acquired after surgery (to the right) in Fig. 11.3. To be able to compare the images they need to be aligned. For that purpose, an operator has placed five corresponding landmarks. They are shown with numbers in the images. We decide that the image taken before operation is the reference image $\mathcal{R}$ and the image taken after is the template image $\mathcal{T}$. The five coordinates, a_i, from the reference image and the five corresponding coordinates, b_i from the template image can be seen in Table 11.1. Using vector representation we have for example $a_3 = [273.75, 299.75]^T$.

We use the transformations described in Chap. 10 to map the landmarks of the reference image to the landmarks of the template image. In this chapter, we introduce a slightly compressed notation. Here the transformation is a function T that takes as input a point $p(x, y)$ and computes the coordinates of the transformed point $p'(x', y')$:

$$p' = T(p),\qquad(11.1)$$

where T can both be a simple transformation (translation or rotation) or a combined transformation involving both scaling, translation, and rotation. The parameters of T depend on the transformation that is used. If it is a simple translation, T has two parameters $(\Delta x, \Delta y)$ and if it is translation and rotation it has three parameters $(\Delta x, \Delta y, \theta)$. T is used to transform all landmarks from the reference image thereby creating a new set of transformed landmarks $a'_i = T(a_i)$. Later it will be explained why we transform the landmarks of the reference image and not the landmarks of the template image.

Our goal is to find the transformation that transforms the landmarks of the reference image so they fit as best as possible to the landmarks of the template image. Basically, it means that the transformed landmarks a'_i should be close to b_i. For that purpose, we define a function that describes how well the two point sets are aligned. A commonly used function is the *sum of squared distances*:

$$F = \sum_{i=1}^{N} D(T(a_i), b_i)^2,\qquad(11.2)$$

where $D(x, y)$ is the Euclidean distance between two points, which is the length of the line connecting the two points (see Eq. B.8 in Appendix B). Conceptually, Eq. 11.2 can be understood like this: transform all landmarks in the reference image using T and put them together with the landmarks from the template image. Draw a line between all matching pairs of landmarks (for example, between a'_3 and b_3). Measure the length of all the N lines and square the lengths individually. Finally, F is the sum of the squared line lengths.

When the transformed reference landmarks are close to the landmarks from the template image, F is low and it is high when the landmarks do not match well. The goal is therefore to compute the parameters of T that makes F as low as possible. F is also called an *objective function* and finding the minimum of F is called an *optimization problem*. If we put the parameters of T into a vector w, the optimization problem can be written formally like this

$$\hat{w} = \arg\min_{w} F,\qquad(11.3)$$

where $\hat{w}$ is the parameter values of T that when put into Eq. 11.2 makes F as small as possible. For a simple translation, the parameter vector of T is $w = (\Delta x, \Delta y)$. One way to find the optimal parameters $\hat{w}$ is to try all possible values of w and finding the set that gives the smallest F. However, this brute-force is very slow and much better methods exist.

It is well known that when a function is at a minimum or maximum the first derivative is equal to zero, $\frac{\partial F}{\partial w} = 0$. This can in many cases be used to derive an analytical expression for the optimal solution $\hat{w}$. In the following a series of different mappings (with different sets of parameters w) will be described.

11.1.1   Translation

If the two images is just moved and not rotated or scaled compared to each other, we only need to care about the translation part of the transformation. A geometrical transformation consisting of a pure translation $t = (\Delta x, \Delta y)$ is (equals Eq. 10.3 in Chap. 10)

$$T\begin{pmatrix} x \\ y \end{pmatrix} = \begin{bmatrix} x \\ y \end{bmatrix} + \begin{bmatrix} \Delta x \\ \Delta y \end{bmatrix}. \tag{11.4}$$

The parameter vector used in Eq. 11.3 is therefore $w = (\Delta x, \Delta y)$. For example, will the transformation of point $a_2 = [110.25, 374.25]^T$ with parameter vector $w = [10, 20]^T$ result in $a_2' = T(a_2) = [120.25, 394.25]^T$.

To find the optimal translation when corresponding landmarks are given, the translation that minimizes F should be computed. For a pure translation, Eq. 11.2 becomes

$$F = \sum_{i=1}^{N} \|(a_i + t) - b_i\|^2, \tag{11.5}$$

where $\|.\|$ is the vector length and therefore equal to D. By differentiation with respect to t and setting equal to zero, it can be shown that the estimated optimal translation is

$$\hat{t} = \bar{b} - \bar{a}, \tag{11.6}$$

where

$$\bar{a} = \frac{1}{N} \sum_{i=1}^{N} a_i \qquad \text{and} \qquad \bar{b} = \frac{1}{N} \sum_{i=1}^{N} b_i. \tag{11.7}$$

This can be seen as an alignment of the centers of masses of the two landmark point clouds. When using Eq. 11.7 with the landmarks from Table 11.1 we obtain $\bar{a} = (285.35, 274.45)$ and $\bar{b} = (268.975, 259.525)$. The optimal translation is therefore $t = (-16.375, -24.925)$. The optimal translation applied to the points from the reference image can be seen in Fig. 11.4.

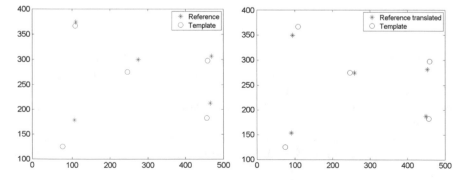

Fig. 11.4 The landmarks from Fig. 11.3. To the left is the unregistered positions. To the right the optimal translation is applied to the points from the reference image

11.1.2   Translation + Rotation = Rigid Transformation

The rigid transformation is often used when we need to compensate for different patients positioning in the same scanner at different times of imaging. That the transformation is rigid, means that there isS no deformation of the image. The rigid transformation consists of a translation $t = (\Delta x, \Delta y)$ and a rotation θ. The parameter vector used in Eq. 11.3 is therefore $w = (\Delta x, \Delta y, \theta)$. The rotation is performed using an orthogonal matrix R (see Eq. 10.5, Chap. 10)

$$R = \begin{bmatrix} \cos\theta & -\sin\theta \\ \sin\theta & \cos\theta \end{bmatrix}. \tag{11.8}$$

The combined transformation is therefore:

$$T\begin{pmatrix} x \\ y \end{pmatrix} = R\begin{bmatrix} x \\ y \end{bmatrix} + t. \tag{11.9}$$

The objective function in Eq. 11.2 becomes

$$F = \sum_{i=1}^{N} \|(Ra_i + t) - b_i\|^2. \tag{11.10}$$

To find the minimum of this objective function a small trick is needed. We introduce the centered landmark sets $\tilde{a}_i = a_i - \bar{a}$ and $\tilde{b}_i = b_i - \bar{b}$. This is equal to translating both point sets so their centers of masses are placed at the origin. In our example, the two landmark sets from Fig. 11.3 have been centered so they are both placed around the origin of the coordinate system, as seen in Fig. 11.5. It can be seen that a small rotation around the origin could probably align them better.

By inserting the centered landmarks in Eq. 11.10, the objective function becomes

$$F = \sum_{i=1}^{N} \|R\tilde{a}_i - \tilde{b}_i + t - (\bar{b} - R\bar{a})\|^2. \tag{11.11}$$

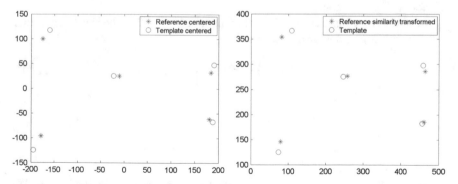

Fig. 11.5 The landmarks from Fig. 11.3. To the left, the two landmark sets have been centered. To the right, the reference landmarks have been aligned with the template landmarks using a similarity transformation

Now the goal is to find the minimum of F. Initially, we differentiate with respect to t. This gives $t = \bar{b} - R\bar{a}$ and inserting this in Eq. 11.11 we obtain

$$
F = \sum_{i=1}^{N} \| R\tilde{a}_i - \tilde{b}_i \|^2
$$

$$
= \sum_{i=1}^{N} \left[\tilde{a}_i^T R^T R\tilde{a}_i + \tilde{b}_i^T \tilde{b}_i - 2\tilde{a}_i^T R^T \tilde{b}_i \right]. \tag{11.12}
$$

Now, using $R^T R = I$ it can be shown[1] [8] that we obtain the minimizing R by performing a so-called singular value decomposition of

$$
H = \sum_{i=1}^{N} \tilde{a}_i \tilde{b}_i^T = UDV^T, \tag{11.13}
$$

with $U^T U = V^T V = I$, and $D = \text{diag}(\lambda_1, \lambda_2, \lambda_3)$ with $\lambda_1 \geq \lambda_2 \geq \lambda_3$—and setting

$$
\hat{R} = V\,\text{diag}(1, 1, \det(VU))U^T
$$

$$
\hat{t} = \bar{b} - \hat{R}\bar{a} \tag{11.14}
$$

The diagonal matrix interposed between V and U ensures that we get a proper rotation, i.e., reflections are avoided.

11.1.3 Translation + Rotation + Isotropic Scaling = Similarity Transformation

The similarity transformation adds isotropic scaling to the rigid transformation. Isotropic scaling means that the scaling is not dependent on direction. This means that in addition to different patients positioning we can also compensate for different spatial resolutions in various imaging modalities, i.e., registering MR to CT images. Also in population studies, we often would like to compensate for different sizes of different patients anatomy.

The similarity adds an isotropic scaling parameter $s > 0$ to the rigid transformation. The resulting transformation becomes

$$
T \begin{pmatrix} x \\ y \end{pmatrix} = sR \begin{bmatrix} x \\ y \end{bmatrix} + t \ . \tag{11.15}
$$

---

[1] As a curiosity we mention that this problem is also called the ordinary Procrustes problem. Procrustes was a character from Greek mythology. He was an innkeeper who having only one guest bed fitted his guests to it by stretching of squeezing them as appropriate. The analogy refers to our "stretching" or "squeezing" of one set of landmarks to fit to the other set.

And the parameter vector $w = (\Delta x, \Delta y, \theta, s)$. Computations similar to those for the rigid transformation yield:

$$\hat{R} = V \operatorname{diag}(1, 1, \det(VU))U^T$$

$$\hat{s} = \frac{\sum_{i=1}^{N} \tilde{a}_i^T \hat{R}^T \tilde{b}_i}{\sum_{i=1}^{N} \tilde{a}_i^T \tilde{a}_i}$$

$$\hat{t} = \bar{b} - \hat{s}\hat{R}\bar{a} \tag{11.16}$$

In Fig. 11.5 to the right, the points from Fig. 11.3 have been aligned using a similarity transformation.

11.1.4 Image Transformation

The result of using one of the algorithms above to estimate the parameters of the transformation T is that we now have a way to transform all pixels in one image to fit with the pixels of the other image. As stated before, T transforms a coordinate in the reference image to a coordinate in the template image. However, we would like to keep the reference image untouched and transform the template image. So why this inverse transformation? The answer is that we want to use the backward mapping approach described in Sect. 10.2. The transformed template image is therefore created by initially creating an empty image with the same dimensions as the reference image. For each pixel in this image, the transformation T is computed and the corresponding point is found in the template image. This point is not necessarily placed exactly on a pixel and therefore bilinear interpolation is used to compute the correct pixel value. This value is now placed in the empty image at the current position. In Fig. 11.6 the result of registration can be seen. Here the second image of the hand has been translated and rotated so the landmarks placed on the hands are as close together as possible.

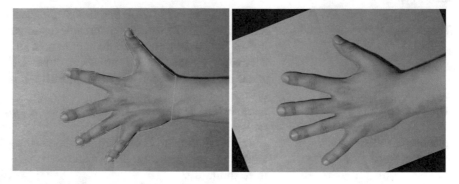

Fig. 11.6 The hands from Fig. 11.2 after the second image of the hand has been translated and rotated such that the sum-of-squared distances between landmarks are minimized

11.2   Intensity-Based Image Registration

The landmark-based method described in the previous section is limited by the fact
that an experienced person is needed to place the landmarks on all images that should
be aligned. Since there is so much information in image, it is obvious to develop
methods that can do the alignment automatically based on the information in the
images. In fact, a large number of algorithms that do exactly that exist. However,
they can be quite advanced and they are considered beyond the scope of this book.
We will, however, introduce the concepts that these methods use.

Normally, we have a reference $\mathcal{R}$ and a template image $\mathcal{T}$. The basic idea is to
move, rotate, and stretch the template image so it fits the reference image as best as
possible. In the previous section, we only looked at simple image transformations
(rigid and similarity). However, often a so-called *spline* transformation is used, where
the template image acts like rubber membrane that can be stretched and compressed
locally. Another important factor is how to compare the reference and the transformed
template image (a similarity measure). A simple method is to subtract the two images
and examine the sum of the differences of the pixel values. This is simple, but not very
robust since the two images could be acquired using different levels of brightness
and contrast (see Sect. 4.1). A better alternative is to use the normalized cross-
correlation as described in Sect. 5.2.1. In fact, image registration is similar to image
template matching with the addition that in image registration the template image
can be transformed in many different ways. It gets even more complicated when the
reference and the template image are not created by the same type of machine. When
comparing a CT image with an MR image the correlation is low, since the different
types of tissues are looking very different on the two types of machine (bone is
white on CT and black on MR, for example). One solution is to use a method called
mutual information to compare the images. We will not go into detail about mutual
information here, but the important point is that the choice of method to compare
the images depends on the type of images that is used.

In summary, intensity-based image registration consists of the following elements [4]:

The geometrical transformation	required to transform the template to the reference image. In some cases a rigid transformation, i.e., a translation and a rotation suffices, in other situations a non-linear geometrical transformation is necessary.
The similarity	measure that describes the goodness of the registration.
The optimization	algorithm that controls (determines the parameters of) the geometrical transformations to maximize similarity.
The regularization	term securing that only reasonable transformations are obtained.

Each of the items listed is a research area in its own right. A great number of different algorithms and methods for each discipline exist.

As with the landmark-based methods, the transform T is described using a set of parameters w. While the rigid transformation is described by three parameters, non-linear transformations (as the spline-based methods) are described using many more parameters. The goal is to find the set of parameters $\hat{w}$, so T transforms the template image so it fits the reference image as best as possible. This can be formulated as

$$\hat{w} = \arg \min_{w} F, \tag{11.17}$$

where the objective function F is formulated as

$$F = S\left(\mathcal{R}, T(\mathcal{T})\right), \tag{11.18}$$

where S is a function that measures similarity between two images (cross-correlation, for example) and $T(\mathcal{T})$ is the template image transformed using T.

Finding $\hat{w}$ is normally not so simple as in the previous section, where equations could be found that gave the optimal solution directly. Instead, a so-called optimization algorithm has to be used. One of the simplest approaches is called the *steepest descent algorithm*. It is based on the idea of finding the gradient vector of F with respect to w. The gradient describes how to change w so F will decrease the most. Optimization is a large topic and we will not pursue it further here.

Finally, a concept called *regularization* is used when advanced transformations are applied to the images. Advanced transformations often have the problem, that they are difficult to control. If the images do not have a very good fit, the transformation will sometimes stretch the template image very much to make it fit the reference image. The result is a stretched template image that no longer is anatomically correct. If, for example, a finger bone is stretched to its double length to make the images fit, something must be wrong. To avoid these types of problem a limit is put onto the transformation. The limit can, for example, be a spring force that makes it proportionally harder for the algorithm to stretch the template image. Using these types of limits is called regularization.

Line and Path Detection

12

The goal of many image analysis algorithms is to recognize a specific pattern in an image. A typical example is face recognition, where a computer has been trained to recognize faces in an image. In this chapter, we focus on two simple and fast approaches to detect two simple patterns in an image, namely, straight lines and curves. Straight lines are detected using the so-called Hough transform and curves are found using an approach based on dynamic programming.

12.1 The Hough Transform

The Hough transform is a powerful tool in image analysis. It was first introduced in 1962 by Paul Hough as a method to recognize particle tracks in a bubble chamber. The purpose of the Hough transform is to detect lines in images. The method has later been extended to more complex shapes like circles and ellipses, but here we will focus on the ability to detect straight lines.

A straight line can be represented in the slope-intercept parameterization:

$$y = ax + b, \qquad (12.1)$$

where a is the slope and b the intercept. However, this is not suitable for all lines. A vertical line cannot be represented by Eq. 12.1, since that would mean that $a = \infty$. This difficulty has lead to the so-called *normal parameterization*, which describes the line by its distance ρ from the origin and the orientation θ of its normal vector:

$$x \cos \theta + y \sin \theta = \rho. \qquad (12.2)$$

This can be seen in Fig. 12.1. The normal parameterization is closely related to the general definition of a line:

© Springer Nature Switzerland AG 2020

R. R. Paulsen and T. B. Moeslund, *Introduction to Medical Image Analysis*,

Undergraduate Topics in Computer Science,

https://doi.org/10.1007/978-3-030-39364-9_12

Fig. 12.1 Normal
parameterisation of a line

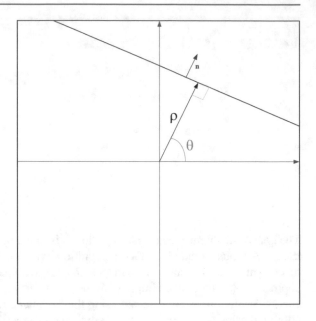

$$Ax + By = C, \tag{12.3}$$

where $A^2 + B^2 = 1$. It is seen that in the normal parameterization $A = \cos\theta$ and $B = \sin\theta$ and therefore the line normal is $\mathbf{n} = (\cos\theta, \sin\theta)$. This can also been seen in Fig. 12.1. Obviously $A^2 + B^2 = (\cos\theta)^2 + (\sin\theta)^2 = 1$. The normal parameterization can easily be transformed into slope-intercept form:

$$y = \left(-\frac{\cos\theta}{\sin\theta}\right)x + \left(\frac{\rho}{\sin\theta}\right). \tag{12.4}$$

The angle θ is restricted to the interval $[0; \pi[$ (or in degrees $[0, 180°]$) so that ρ can be both positive and negative. In the following, we will consider lines in an image where the origin is in the center of the image. The maximum distance from the origin to a pixel in the image is

$$R = \frac{1}{2}\sqrt{W^2 + H^2}, \tag{12.5}$$

where W is the width and H the height of the image (in pixels). The distance parameter ρ in Eq. 12.2 is therefore restricted to $[-R, R]$.

An arbitrary line in an image can now be described by a couple of parameters (ρ, θ). This parameter can also be seen as a point in *Hough Space*. Hough Space is a two-dimensional coordinate system, where ρ is on the vertical axis and θ is on the horizontal axis. Three lines defined in the normal parametrization are seen together with their Hough Space coordinates are shown in Fig. 12.2.

In the following, the practical use of the Hough space is described. In Fig. 12.3 it can be seen how the edges of the metacarpal bones have been found. There are no clear straight lines, but the borders of the bones still follow an approximate line. In Fig. 12.3 to the right, three straight line segments have been marked. Each of them

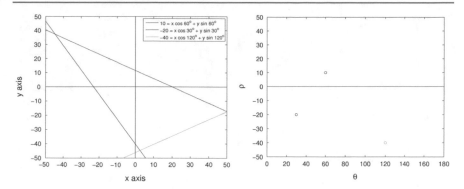

Fig. 12.2 Left: Three lines in the normalized parameterisation. Right: Hough Space with the three lines seen as points

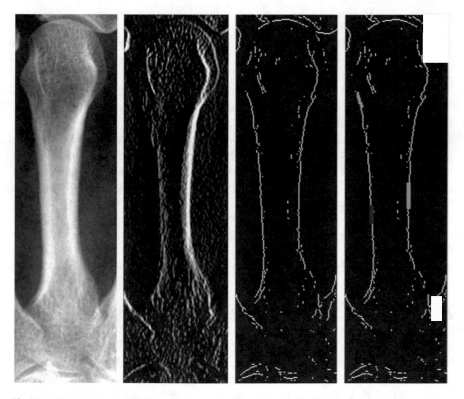

Fig. 12.3 From left to right: X-ray of a metacarpal bone, Prewitt filtered to enhance bone boundaries, significant edges detected, three line segments marked

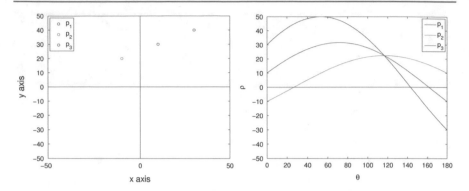

Fig. 12.4 Left: Three points lying on a line candidate. Right: The resulting three sinusoidal curves in Hough Space

corresponds to a point in Hough space. Imagine that all straight line segments in the image were identified and their corresponding points in Hough space were marked. The result would be a collection of points, where some points would be gathered in clusters. Each cluster would correspond to an approximate line in the input image. The problem would now be to identify the clusters in Hough space. However, this is quite difficult and therefore an alternative approach is used.

The essential idea in the Hough transform is that a given point that might lie on a line in an image is mapped to all points in the $\rho - \theta$ parameter space that specify a possible line through the point. If a potential line point has the coordinates (x_l, y_l) in the image, Eq. 12.2 can be used to compute all the points in the Hough space that correspond to potential lines in the image. By computing all ρ values for $\theta \in [0, \pi[$ using $\rho = x_l \cos \theta + y_l \sin \theta$ a sinusoidal curve will be created. The three sinusoidal curves responding to three points that could lie on a line are seen in Fig. 12.4. The three lines are collinear (they lie on a line) and therefore the three sinusoidal curves meet at one point. The (ρ, θ)-coordinates of this point is exactly the parameters of the line going through the three points.

A quantized version of the Hough space is now created. It is represented as a two-dimensional array $\mathbf{H}(l, k)$ of size M x N. This means that the values of θ are sampled $\theta_l = l \cdot \Delta\theta$, where $\Delta\theta = \pi/M$. Consequently, ρ is quantized $\rho_k = -R + k \cdot \Delta\rho$, where $\Delta\rho = 2 \cdot R/N$. The array $\mathbf{H}(l, k)$ can be regarded as a digital image, that are indexed by $l \in [0, \ldots, M - 1]$ and $k \in [0, \ldots, N - 1]$. Each *pixel* in $\mathbf{H}$ corresponds to a line in the input image and it is therefore possible to generate $M \cdot N$ different lines based on $\mathbf{H}$. In the actual transform, $\mathbf{H}$ is used in a voting scheme, where it keeps track of *votes* on the lines found in the input image. Consider a single pixel detected as an edge pixel, for example, one of the blue edges pixels seen in Fig. 12.3 to the right. This pixel (x_e, y_e) is now used to vote for all the potential lines going through it:

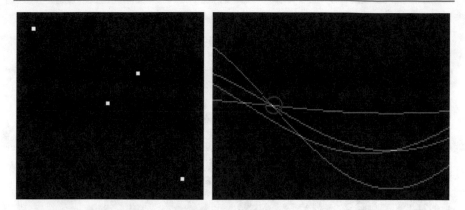

Fig. 12.5 Left: Image with four points detected as potential line points. Right: The resulting quantized Hough space **H** (with θ on the horizontal axis and ρ on the vertical axis). The pixel in Hough space with most votes is shown with the red circle

for $l = 0$ to $M - 1$ **do**

$\qquad \theta_l = l \cdot \Delta\theta$
$\qquad$ Calculate $\rho_k = x_e \cos\theta_l + y_e \sin\theta_l$
$\qquad$ Round ρ_k to the closest value, so $\rho_k = -R + k \cdot \Delta\rho$, where k is an integer.
$\qquad$ Add one to $\mathbf{H}(k, l)$

end for

The above procedure is performed for each pixel that can be considered as lying on a line. In Fig. 12.5 a simple image with four points identified as edge points is seen together with the resulting quantized Hough space **H**. The pixel with the most accumulated votes is shown with a red circle. It corresponds to the line going through the three collinear points.

The most prominent lines in the input image can therefore be identified by searching for the pixel in Hough space with the most votes. A typical procedure is to first find the pixel with the highest value and then set all pixels in its neighborhood (radius 3 for example) to zero and then find the next highest pixel and so on. This process continues until a threshold in votes is met or a fixed number of lines have been found. In Fig. 12.6 the Hough space for the metacarpal edge image is shown together with the two lines that correspond to the two highest peaks in **H**. Usually, the found lines extend to infinity, but for visual purposes only the part that overlaps the edge is shown on the figure.

Finally, the complete Hough transform can be summed up. Start by creating an edge filtered version of the input image **I**. The result is a binary image $\mathbf{I}_e$, where a value of 1 indicates that this pixel is a potential line pixel. An example can be seen in Fig. 12.3. The Hough space **H** is then computed by

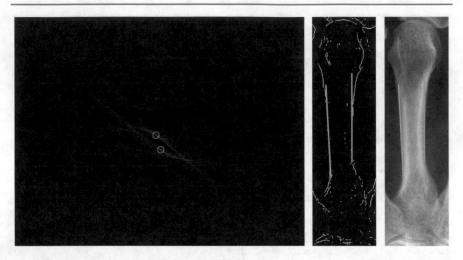

Fig. 12.6 Left: Hough space of edges in metacarpal image with two maxima shown with green circles. Middle: Found lines shown on edge image. Right: Found lines on original image

for each pixel (x, y) in $\mathbf{I}_e$ **do**

    if $\mathbf{I}_e(x, y) > 0$ **then**

        for $l = 0$ to $M - 1$ **do**

            $\theta_l = l \cdot \Delta\theta$
            Calculate $\rho_k = x_e \cos\theta_l + y_e \sin\theta_l$
            Round ρ_k to the closest value, so $\rho_k = -R + k \cdot \Delta\rho$, where k is an integer.
            Add one to $\mathbf{H}(k, l)$

        end for

    end if

end for

The parameters of the line candidates are now found as maxima in $\mathbf{H}$.

There are several ways that the Hough transform can be made faster and many extensions exist.

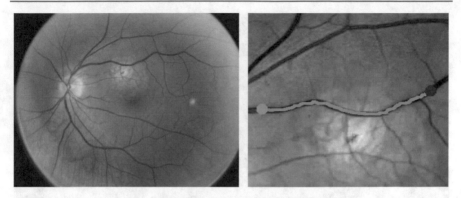

Fig. 12.7 To the left is seen a photograph of the fundus of the eye. The dark lines are arteries and veins and the bright spot is the optic cup. To the right one of the veins has been tracked using dynamic programming

12.2 Path Tracing Using Dynamic Programming

A very useful tool in image analysis is the ability to recognize and track edges or boundaries in images. In the following, a path can both be a boundary between different organs, a curved line, or another anatomical feature that can be described using a piecewise linear function. An example can be seen in Fig. 12.7, where the goal is to track the veins in the eye. Using a special technique called *fundus photography* it is possible to acquire images of the human fundus. Several disorders, including diabetes, can be diagnosed based on the appearance of the veins and arteries seen in a fundus photograph. To the right in Fig. 12.7, a path has been tracked from the red dot to the green dot. In the following, a method that can be used to compute optimal paths is described.

A path algorithm finds an optimal path from one point to another. A typical example is a GPS device that calculates the route going from one city to another. Inside the device, a list of all cities is stored together with the distances between all neighboring cities. This data structure is also called a *graph*, where the cities are *nodes* and the roads between the cities are *edges*.[1] The shortest path algorithm computes the path that will bring you from one city to another using the least amount of gasoline (or the least amount of time or traveled distance).

A commonly used algorithm is *Dijkstra's algorithm* that is based on *dynamic programming*.[2] In Dijkstra's algorithm, one node is selected and called the *source* and the algorithm then computes the shortest path to all other nodes in the graph. It

---

[1] Sometimes a node is called a *vertex* and an edge is called a *line*.

[2] Dynamic programming does not mean programming of computers, but is actually a synonym for *optimisation*.

140	190	73	19	60
130	212	14	100	145
150	20	80	135	120
157	140	33	199	100
121	234	45	210	86

140	190	73	19	60
130	212	14	100	145
150	20	80	135	120
157	140	33	199	100
121	234	45	210	86

Fig. 12.8 To the left an image, **I**, used as input in a pathfinding algorithm. To the right the possible directions a path can take from a single pixel

is therefore also called a single-source shortest path algorithm. In the following, a simplified version of Dijkstra's algorithm is described.

Consider an image **I**, where each pixel has a value between 0 and 255. A cost function $C(r, c)$ is now defined that returns the cost of entering a pixel at position (r, c) in the image. Initially, the cost is defined as being the same as the pixel value. In the image seen in Fig. 12.8 the cost of entering the pixel at $(2, 3)$ is $C(2, 3) = 14$. It is convenient to think of a car driving around on the image, where the pixel values are the height of the terrain. It will then cost 14 units of gasoline to drive from a neighbor pixel into the pixel at $(2, 3)$.

We now limit ourselves to search for an optimal path $\mathcal{P}$ going from the top to the bottom of the image. The optimal path is defined as the path with the lowest accumulated cost:

$$C_{\text{tot}} = \sum_{(r,c)\in\mathcal{P}} C(r, c), \qquad (12.6)$$

The path is defined as a list of the (r, c) coordinates of the pixel in the path. For the image in Fig. 12.8 one path could be $\mathcal{P} = [(1, 3), (2, 3), (3, 2), (4, 3), (5, 4)]$. This path has the accumulated cost of $C_{\text{tot}} = 73 + 14 + 20 + 33 + 210 = 350$.

Obviously, the optimal path can be found by calculating C_{tot} for all possible paths going from the top to the bottom of the image. However, even for small images, this would require huge amounts of calculations. Dynamic programming is a way to overcome this by breaking large problems into smaller and more manageable subproblems. As a start, we limit ourselves to paths that for each step can either go straight down one pixel, one pixel down to the left, and one pixel down to the right as seen in Fig. 12.8 to the right. The algorithm starts by creating two images with the same dimensions as the input image. The first is called the *accumulator image* **A** and the second is called the *backtracing image* **T**. The accumulator image is used

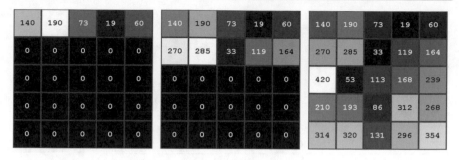

Fig. 12.9 The accumulator image **A**. Left: Before first iterations. Middle: After first iteration. Right: After all iterations

to keep track of the accumulated cost when moving down the input image and the backtracing image keeps track of the possible paths through the input image.

Initially, the first row of pixel values from the input image is copied to the accumulator image as seen in Fig. 12.9 to the left. In the first iteration of the algorithm, the second row of the accumulator image is updated. For each pixel in this row, the three pixels above are inspected (straight up, left-up, and right-up) and the one with the lowest value is selected. This is the lowest possible cost to go to the current pixel from the top of the image. The current pixel in the accumulator image is now set to this value added with the current value in the input image. Formally,

$$\mathbf{A}(r, c) = \mathbf{I}(r, c) + \min\left(\mathbf{A}(r - 1, c - 1), \mathbf{A}(r - 1, c), \mathbf{A}(r - 1, c + 1)\right), \quad (12.7)$$

where $\mathbf{A}(r - 1, c)$ is the pixel just above in the accumulator image, $\mathbf{A}(r - 1, c - 1)$ is the left-up pixel and $\mathbf{A}(r - 1, c + 1)$ is the right-up pixel. The pixel at position $(r, c) = (2, 3)$ has the value $I(2, 3) = 14$ in the input image and $\min(190, 73, 19) = 19$ therefore $\mathbf{A}(2, 3) = 33$. So the lowest possible cost to go from the top of the image down to the pixel at $(2, 3)$ is 33. The accumulator image after the first row has been processed can be seen in Fig. 12.9 in the middle.

The algorithm continues, by repeating the process for the next row until the end of the image. The accumulator image after all iterations can be seen in Fig. 12.9 to the right.[3] The endpoint of the optimal path is now chosen as the pixel in **A** with the lowest value on the last row. The value of this pixel gives the exact cost of the cheapest way of going from the top to the bottom of the image. This is the same as the optimal cost from Eq. 12.6. As seen in Fig. 12.9 to the right, $C_{\text{tot}} = 131$.

We know now what the accumulated cost is for the optimal path, but we did not keep track of the path when calculating the cost. To find the path, a technique known as *backtracing* is used. During the iterations, the backtracing image **T** is used to keep track of potential paths. When **A** is updated using Eq. 12.7 the column number of the pixel with the lowest value is stored in **T**. Consider the pixel at position $(2, 3)$. It was seen earlier that the accumulated cost at that pixel is $\mathbf{A}(2, 3) =$

---

[3]The input image is padded with values of 255.

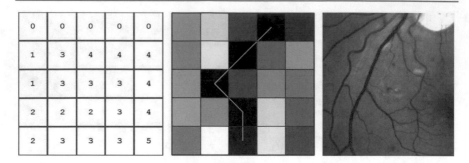

Fig. 12.10 Left: The final backtracing image **T**. Middle: The found path drawn on the input image. Right: Path tracing on an extracted part of a fundus image

$I(2, 3) + A(1, 4) = 33$. The path going down to that pixel would therefore *come* from the pixel at $(r, c) = (1, 4)$ and as a result $\mathbf{T}(2, 3) = 4$.

Finally, the path can be tracked by starting at the pixel with the lowest accumulated cost in the last row of **A**. In the example, this is $(5, 3)$. The value of $\mathbf{T}(5, 3) = 3$ tells us that the next path entry is $(4, 3)$. Here the value of $\mathbf{T}(4, 3) = 2$ gives the next step $(3, 2)$. Finally, the optimal path is found to be $\mathcal{P} = [(1, 4), (2, 3), (3, 2), (4, 3), (5, 3)]$, where the order is reversed so the path goes from the top to the bottom of the image. It can be seen in the middle on Fig. 12.10.

The algorithm has been tested on an extracted part of a fundus image as seen in Fig. 12.10 to the right. The found path follows the major vein with a few perturbations. The image is acquired and preprocessed so the veins appear dark on a bright background, which makes the image suitable for path processing. However, it is not always the case that the structures that should be followed appear as dark lines on a bright background. In the following sections, we will demonstrate how preprocessing can be used to create suitable input for the path tracing algorithm.

12.2.1 Preprocessing for Path Tracing

The described approach to finding paths in images can easily be adapted and made more versatile. In the previous section, it was used to find dark lines in images. In Fig. 12.11 to the left, the ulna and radius bones as seen on arm X-ray photographs are shown. We would like to estimate the bone thickness and the first step is to compute the outer borders of the bones. The anatomical border between the bone and the soft-tissue is not a dark line, but is characterized by a sharp gradient in the pixel values. An intuitive approach is therefore to turn the highest gradients in the image into the darkest path. This can be done by filtering the input image with a gradient filter as seen in Fig. 12.11 middle. Here the gradients are approximated by first computing a smoothed image $\mathbf{I}_G$ using a Gaussian filter kernel (here size $[11 \times 11]$). The gradient image is then $\mathbf{I}_\Delta = \mathbf{I}_G - \mathbf{I}_G^+$, where $\mathbf{I}_G^+$ is the smoothed image translated one pixel to the right. The inverse of the gradient image will naturally have dark lines, where

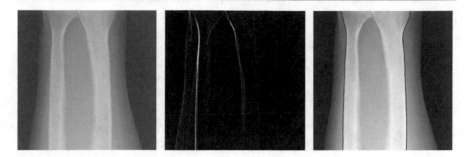

Fig. 12.11 Left: The ulna and radius bone seen on an X-ray of a human arm. Middle: The result of a gradient-based filter on the input image. Right: The outer limits of the radius and ulna found using dynamic programming

there are high gradients in the input image. The cost function used in the path finding is therefore $C(r, c) = -\mathbf{I}_\Delta(r, c)$. In our case, the function is simplified to

$$C(r, c) = -(\mathbf{I}_G(r, c) - \mathbf{I}_G(r, c + 1)) . \tag{12.8}$$

In Fig. 12.11 to the right, the result can be seen where the gradients have been computed as in Eq. 12.8 combined with the result from using gradients based on $-(\mathbf{I}_G(r, c + 1) - \mathbf{I}_G(r, c))$. The method locates the outer border of both bones successfully. Experience shows that it is harder to locate the inner borders of both bones. This is due to the cross-sectional shape of the bone that is tear-shaped. The gradients caused by the inner borders are therefore weaker than the gradients caused by the outer borders.

12.2.2   Locating Circular Structures

The simple path tracing algorithm described in the early section can be adapted further and applied to more complex problem. An example is seen in Fig. 12.12 to the left, where some organs can be seen on an abdominal CT scan. We are interested in automatically computing the boundary between the left kidney and the surrounding tissue. This is a closed circular structure and in the following it is explained how the simple path tracer can be adapted to these type of structures. Initially, a midpoint (r_m, c_m) is selected manually, as seen as the red dot to the right in Fig. 12.12. From this midpoint a set of *spokes*[4] are computed. In Fig. 12.12 to the right, a set of $N = 36$ spokes are shown. One spoke is defined by a start point $(r_s, c_s) = (r_m, c_m)$ and an endpoint (r_e, c_e). The endpoints for all spokes are found as

$$r_e = r_s + \cos(\theta) \cdot L$$
$$c_e = c_s + \sin(\theta) \cdot L,$$

---

[4]Think of spokes in an old fashioned wheel.

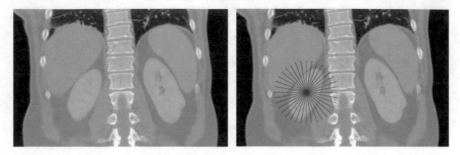

Fig. 12.12 Left: CT scan of the abdominal area. Right: An example of how the image can be resampled. The red dot is the manually selected middle point

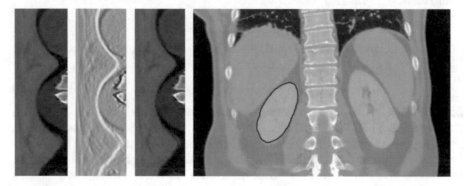

Fig. 12.13 From left to right: Resampled image using 360 spokes, gradient filter applied to the resampled image, the path found in the resampled image, the path on the input image

where L is the length of the spoke and $\theta = \frac{2\pi n}{N}, n = [0, 1, \ldots, N-1]$. A *resampled* version of the input image is created by sampling the pixel values under the spokes and using them to create a new image. The pixel samples for the spoke with $n = 0$ will constitute the first row of the new image, and the pixel sampled using the spoke with $n = N - 1$ will be the last row. A resampled image can be seen in Fig. 12.13. When sampling the spokes in the input image, the sampling positions are not normally consistent with the exact pixel positions in the input image and therefore a pixel interpolation method like bi-linear or bi-cubic interpolation should be used.

The resampled image can now be used as input to the path approach described in the previous image. A gradient image is computed based on the resampled image, to force the path to follow high gradients in the image. The gradient image can be seen in Fig. 12.13. The simple path tracing algorithm can now be applied to the inverse of the gradient image. A result can be seen in Fig. 12.13. Finally, the path can be transformed back to the original image. If a point on the path in the resampled image is (r_p^r, c_p^r), then the position of the point in the input image is

$$r_p^I = r_s + \cos(\theta_p) \cdot c_p^r$$
$$c_p^I = c_s + \sin(\theta_p) \cdot c_p^r,$$

where $\theta_p = \frac{2\pi r_p^r}{N}$. The found path transformed back to the input image can be seen in Fig. 12.13 to the right.

This method can be extended in several ways. A popular approach that is sometimes called *magic scissors* is to initially annotate a sparse set of points on the anatomical boundary followed by a resampling of the image following the lines connecting the annotated points. Dynamic programming is then used to find the optimal path in the resampled image and the path is finally transformed back to the input image.

Appendix
Bits, Bytes, and Binary Numbers

A

When working with images it is useful to know something about how data is stored in the memory of the computer. Most values associated with images are closely related to the internal representation of the numbers. The value of one pixel is often stored as one byte for example.

The memory of the computer can basically be seen as an enormous amount of switches that can either be turned on and off. Each switch is called a bit (binary digit) and can therefore be assigned either the value 0 or the value 1. So if you just wanted to store values of either 0 or 1 it would be perfectly fine. However, this is rarely the case and bits are combined to represent other types of numbers.

Eight bits together are called a byte. With eight bit the total number of different combinations that can be is $2^8 = 256$ and therefore a byte is defined to have values from 0 to 255 (256 values in total). A byte is shown as a row of eight bits (having values 0 or 1). The bit to the left is called the most-significant bit (MSB) and the bit to the right the less-significant bit (LSB). Number represented using bits are called binary numbers. The binary number system is also called a base-2 system, since the basic unit only has two values. Our *normal* system is a base-10 system and is called the decimal system. Some example byte values are as follows:

Binary	Decimal
00000001	1
00000010	2
00000100	4
00000101	5
00001111	15
00010101	21
01010101	85
10000000	128

Sometimes bytes are also appended to create numbers larger than 255. A common example is two bytes together that spans the values $0 - 65535$ ($2^{16} = 65536$ in total).

© Springer Nature Switzerland AG 2020

R. R. Paulsen and T. B. Moeslund, *Introduction to Medical Image Analysis*,
Undergraduate Topics in Computer Science,
https://doi.org/10.1007/978-3-030-39364-9_A

A.1   Conversion from Decimal to Binary

A simple routine exists for getting the binary representation of a decimal number. Initially, the largest power of two that is less than the decimal number is found. If the decimal number is 137, then the largest power of two is 128. This is then subtracted from the original number and the corresponding bit is set. This is repeated until the decimal number is reduced to zero. In our example, 137 is found to be a sum of 128, 8, and 1 and therefore the binary representation of 137 is 10001001.

A.2   Conversion from Binary to Decimal

The conversion from the binary representation to a decimal number is straightforward. The individual bit values are simply added together. The binary number 01100101 consists of active bits with values 64, 32, 4, and 1 and therefore the decimal number is 101.

Appendix
Mathematical Definitions

B

This appendix provides some basic mathematical definitions. The appendix is intended for readers who do not have a mathematical background or readers who need a "brush-up".

B.1 Absolute Value

The *absolute value* of a number, z, is written as $Abs(z)$ or $|z|$. It is calculated by deleting the "minus" in front of the number. This means that $|-150| = 150$. Mathematically the absolute value of a number, z, is calculated as

$$|z| = \sqrt{z^2} \tag{B.1}$$

In terms of programming it can be written as

Implementation of absolute value

```
if (z < 0)
    z = -1 * z;
```

B.2 min and max

The *min* value of a set of numbers is written as $\min\{x_1, x_2, \ldots, x_n\}$ and simply means the smallest number in the set. For example, $\min\{7, 3, 11, 2, 42\} = 2$. The *max* value of a set of numbers is written as $\max\{x_1, x_2, \ldots, x_n\}$ and simply means the biggest number in the set. For example, $\max\{7, 3, 11, 2, 42\} = 42$. In terms of programming the max operation can be written as follows, where we assume that N numbers are present in the list and that they are stored in `list[]`:

© Springer Nature Switzerland AG 2020
R. R. Paulsen and T. B. Moeslund, *Introduction to Medical Image Analysis*,
Undergraduate Topics in Computer Science,
https://doi.org/10.1007/978-3-030-39364-9_B

Table B.1 Different rational numbers and three different ways of converting to integers

x	Floor of x	Ceiling of x	Round of x
3.14	3	4	3
0.7	0	1	1
4.5	4	5	5
−3.14	−4	−3	−3
−0.7	−1	0	−1
−4.5	−5	−4	−4

Implementation of the max operation

```
MaxValue=list[0];
for (i = 1; i < N; i = i+1) {
    if (list[i] > MaxValue)
        MaxValue = list[i];
}
```

B.3 Converting a Rational Number to an Integer

Sometimes we want to convert a rational number into an integer. This can be done in different ways, where the three most common are

Floor simply rounds a rational number to the nearest smaller integer. For example: Floor of 4.2 = 4. Mathematically it is denoted $\lfloor 4.2 \rfloor = 4$. In C-programming a build-in function exists $floor()$

Ceiling is the opposite of floor and rounds off to the nearest bigger integer. For example: Ceiling of 4.2 = 5. Mathematically it is denoted $\lceil 4.2 \rceil = 5$. In C-programming a build-in function exists $ceil()$

Round finds the nearest integer, i.e., Round of 4.2 = 4 and Round of 4.7 = 5. In terms of C-code the following expression is often used: $int(x + 0.5)$. That is, we add 0.5 to the number and then typecast it to an integer.

In Table B.1 some examples are provided.

B.4 Summation

Say you want to add the first 12 positive integers:

$$1 + 2 + 3 + 4 + 5 + 6 + 7 + 8 + 9 + 10 + 11 + 12 = 78 \qquad \text{(B.2)}$$

This is no problem writing down, but what if you want to add the first 1024 positive integers? This will be dreadful to write down. Luckily there exists a more compact way of writing this using *summation*, which is denoted as $\sum$. Adding the first 1024 positive integers can now be written as

$$\sum_{i=1}^{1024} i \ , \qquad \text{(B.3)}$$

where i is the summation index. Below the summation sign we have $i = 1$, which means that the first value of i is 1. Above the summation sign we have 1024. This actually means $i = 1042$, but we virtually always skip $i =$. Either way, it means that the last value of i is 1042. You can think of i as a counter going from 1 to 1042 in steps of one: $1, 2, 3, 4, 5, \ldots, 1040, 1041, 1042$. What comes after the summation is a function, which is controlled by i and it is the values of this function (for each i) that are added together. Below, some examples of different summations are given:

$$\sum_{i=1}^{12} i = 1 + 2 + 3 + 4 + 5 + 6 + 7 + 8 + 9 + 10 + 11 + 12 = 78$$

$$\sum_{i=0}^{4} 2 \cdot i = 0 + 2 + 4 + 6 + 8 = 20$$

$$\sum_{i=-2}^{1} i^2 = 4 + 1 + 0 + 1 = 6$$

Say that you want to sum the pixel values of the first row in an image with width $= 200$. This is then written as

$$\sum_{i=0}^{199} f(i, 0) \qquad \text{(B.4)}$$

In general the summation is written as

$$\sum_{i=n}^{m} h(i) \qquad \text{(B.5)}$$

In terms of C-programming the summation is implemented as a *for-loop*:

Implementation of summation

```
Result=0;
for (i = n; i < (m+1); i = i+1)
{
    Result = Result + h(i);
}
```

We can also do a summation using more indexes than i. For example, if we want to add all pixel values in an image, then we need two indexes representing rows and columns. Concretely we would write

$$\sum_{j=0}^{M-1} \sum_{i=0}^{N-1} f(i, j) \, , \tag{B.6}$$

where N is the number of columns and M is the number of rows. In terms of C-programming the double summation is implemented as two *for-loops*:

Implementation of the double summation

```
Result=0;
for (j = 0; j < M; j = j+1)
{
    for (i = 0; i < N; i=i+1)
    {
        Result = Result + GetPixel(input, i, j);
    }
}
```

B.5 Vector

In the 2D coordinate system in Fig. B.1 a point is defined as $P(x_1, y_1)$. The same point can be represented as a *vector* (as seen in Fig. B.1):

$$\vec{p} = \begin{bmatrix} x_1 \\ y_1 \end{bmatrix} \tag{B.7}$$

A vector is often written as a lowercase letter with an arrow above. It can be interpreted as a line with a slope $\frac{y_1}{x_1}$ and a length. The *length of the vector* is defined as

$$\| \vec{p} \| = \sqrt{x_1^2 + y_1^2} \tag{B.8}$$

We can arrange the vector as a row (as opposed to a column) by taking the *transpose* of the vector, $\vec{p}^T$. That is

$$\vec{p}^T = [x_1 \quad y_1] \tag{B.9}$$

or in other words:

$$\begin{bmatrix} x_1 \\ y_1 \end{bmatrix}^T = [x_1 \quad y_1] \qquad\qquad [x_1 \quad y_1]^T = \begin{bmatrix} x_1 \\ y_1 \end{bmatrix} \tag{B.10}$$

Say we have two vectors: $\vec{p_1}^T = [5 \quad 5]$ and $\vec{p_2}^T = [2 \quad 0]$. We can then calculate the sum of $\vec{p_1}$ and $\vec{p_2}$ as

$$\vec{p_3} = \vec{p_1} + \vec{p_2} = \begin{bmatrix} 5 \\ 5 \end{bmatrix} + \begin{bmatrix} 2 \\ 0 \end{bmatrix} = \begin{bmatrix} 5+2 \\ 5+0 \end{bmatrix} = \begin{bmatrix} 7 \\ 5 \end{bmatrix} . \tag{B.11}$$

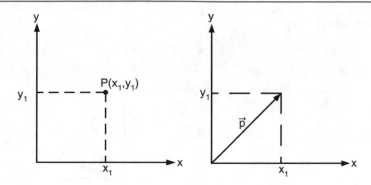

Fig. B.1 Left: Point representation. Right: Vector representation

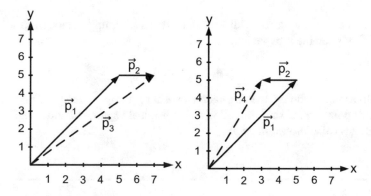

Fig. B.2 Left: Adding two vectors. Right: Subtracting two vectors

In the same way we can calculate the difference of $\vec{p_1}$ and $\vec{p_2}$ as

$$\vec{p_4} = \vec{p_1} - \vec{p_2} = \begin{bmatrix} 5 \\ 5 \end{bmatrix} - \begin{bmatrix} 2 \\ 0 \end{bmatrix} = \begin{bmatrix} 5-2 \\ 5-0 \end{bmatrix} = \begin{bmatrix} 3 \\ 5 \end{bmatrix} \tag{B.12}$$

These operations can also be interpreted geometrically as illustrated in Fig. B.2.

Two vectors cannot be multiplied but we can calculate the *dot product* between them. Say we define $\vec{p_1} = [a \ \ b]^T$ and $\vec{p_2} = [c \ \ d]^T$. The dot product between them is then defined as

$$\vec{p_1} \bullet \vec{p_2} = ac + bd \tag{B.13}$$

The dot product can also be interpreted geometrically as

$$\vec{p_1} \bullet \vec{p_2} = \|\vec{p_1}\| \cdot \|\vec{p_2}\| \cdot \cos V \tag{B.14}$$

where $\|\vec{p_1}\|$ is the length of vector $\vec{p_1}$, $\|\vec{p_2}\|$ is the length of vector $\vec{p_2}$, and V is the angle between the vectors, see Fig. B.3. Note that it is always the smallest of the two possible angles that is calculated using Eq. B.14, i.e., $0° \leq V \leq 180°$. The biggest angle is found as $V_{\text{big}} = 360° - V$

Fig. B.3 The angle between
two vectors

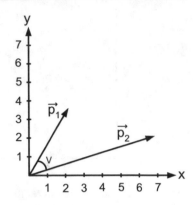

A *unit vector* is a vector with length 1. To create a unit vector from a normal vector $\vec{v}$, you divide it by its length:

$$\vec{u} = \frac{\vec{v}}{\|\vec{v}\|}, \tag{B.15}$$

where division is done by dividing each element of $\vec{v}$ by the length. The result is a vector that points in the same direction as the original vector, but with length 1. This is sometimes called *normalization*.

B.6 Matrix

When we have multiple vectors we can represent them as one entity denoted a *matrix*. For example, $\vec{p_1} = [a \ \ b]^T$ and $\vec{p_2} = [c \ \ d]^T$ can be represented as

$$\mathbf{P} = \begin{bmatrix} a & c \\ b & d \end{bmatrix} \tag{B.16}$$

A matrix is often denoted by an uppercase letter in boldface, but other representations can also be used. To avoid confusion a textbook involving vectors and matrices therefore often contains a preface stating how vectors and matrices are defined.

We say a matrix has a vertical and horizontal dimension, e.g., $\mathbf{P}$ has dimension 2×2. Note that the dimensions need not be equal. Similar to a vector a matrix can also be transposed by making the columns into rows:

$$\mathbf{P}^T = \begin{bmatrix} a & b \\ c & d \end{bmatrix} \tag{B.17}$$

Matrices can be added and subtracted similar to vectors, but they need to have the same dimensions:

$$\begin{bmatrix} a & c \\ b & d \end{bmatrix} + \begin{bmatrix} e & g \\ f & h \end{bmatrix} = \begin{bmatrix} a+e & c+g \\ b+f & d+h \end{bmatrix} \tag{B.18}$$

$$\begin{bmatrix} a & c \\ b & d \end{bmatrix} - \begin{bmatrix} e & g \\ f & h \end{bmatrix} = \begin{bmatrix} a-e & c-g \\ b-f & d-h \end{bmatrix} \tag{B.19}$$

Matrices can be multiplied in the following way:

$$\begin{bmatrix} a & c \\ b & d \end{bmatrix} \cdot \begin{bmatrix} e & g \\ f & h \end{bmatrix} = \begin{bmatrix} ae + cf & ag + ch \\ be + df & bg + dh \end{bmatrix} \tag{B.20}$$

The entry in row one and column one of the output matrix $(ae + cf)$ is found as the dot product between row one of the left matrix and column one of the right matrix. This principle is then repeated for each entry in the output matrix. This implies that the number of columns in the left matrix has to be equal to the number of rows in the right matrix. On the other hand, this also implies that the number of rows in the left matrix and the number of columns in the right matrix need not be the same. For example, a matrix can be multiplied by a vector. The dimensions of the output matrix are equal to the number of rows in the left matrix and the number of columns in the right matrix. Below, some examples are shown:

$$\mathbf{A} \cdot \mathbf{B} = \mathbf{C} \tag{B.21}$$
$$(3 \times 2) \cdot (2 \times 7) = (3 \times 7)$$
$$(12 \times 3) \cdot (3 \times 1) = (12 \times 1)$$

A matrix of particular interest is the *identity matrix*, which in the 2D case looks like this:

$$\mathbf{I} = \begin{bmatrix} 1 & 0 \\ 0 & 1 \end{bmatrix} \tag{B.22}$$

If the product of two matrices equals the identity matrix, $\mathbf{A} \cdot \mathbf{B} = \mathbf{I}$, then we say they are each other's *inverse*. This is denoted as $\mathbf{A}^{-1} = \mathbf{B}$ and $\mathbf{B}^{-1} = \mathbf{A}$, or in other words $\mathbf{A} \cdot \mathbf{A}^{-1} = \mathbf{A}^{-1} \cdot \mathbf{A} = \mathbf{I}$. For a 2×2 matrix the inverse is calculated as

$$\begin{bmatrix} a & c \\ b & d \end{bmatrix}^{-1} = \frac{1}{ad - bc} \cdot \begin{bmatrix} d & -c \\ -b & a \end{bmatrix} \tag{B.23}$$

Calculating the inverse for matrices of higher dimensions can be quite complicated. For further information see a textbook on linear algebra.

B.7 Applying Linear Algebra

Say you want to find the equation of a straight line $y = \alpha x + \beta$. You know that the line passes through the point $P_1(x, y) = (2, 3)$, so we have that $3 = 2\alpha + \beta$. Obviously, this is not enough information to find α and β, or in other words we have one equation and two unknowns α and β. So in order to solve the problem we need to know the coordinates of one more point on the line or in other words we need two equations to find two unknowns. Say that we then have another point on the line, $P_2(x, y) = (1, 1)$, yielding $1 = \alpha + \beta$, we can solve the problem in the following manner. From the last equation we can see that $\alpha = 1 - \beta$. If we insert this into the first equation we get $3 = 2(1 - \beta) + \beta \Leftrightarrow \beta = -1$ and from this follows that $\alpha = 2$. So the equation for the line is $y = 2x - 1$. This principle can be used to solve simple problems where we have a few equations and a few unknowns. But imagine we have 10 equations with 10 unknowns, that would require quite an effort (and most likely we would make mistakes along the way). Instead, we can use linear algebra and get the computer to help us.

Using linear algebra to solve these kinds of problems is carried out by arranging the equations into the form: $\vec{a} = \mathbf{B} \cdot \vec{c}$, where $\vec{a}$ and $\mathbf{B}$ are known and $\vec{c}$ contains the unknowns. The solution is then found by multiplying by the inverse of $\mathbf{B}$:

$$\vec{a} = \mathbf{B} \cdot \vec{c} \qquad\qquad \Leftrightarrow \qquad\qquad \text{(B.24)}$$

$$\mathbf{B}^{-1}\vec{a} = \mathbf{B}^{-1}\mathbf{B} \cdot \vec{c} \qquad\qquad \Leftrightarrow \qquad\qquad \text{(B.25)}$$

$$\mathbf{B}^{-1}\vec{a} = \mathbf{I} \cdot \vec{c} \qquad\qquad \Leftrightarrow \qquad\qquad \text{(B.26)}$$

$$\mathbf{B}^{-1}\vec{a} = \vec{c} \qquad\qquad\qquad\qquad \text{(B.27)}$$

For the example with the two lines we have

$$\begin{matrix} 3 = 2\alpha + \beta \\ 1 = \alpha + \beta \end{matrix} \Rightarrow \begin{bmatrix} 3 \\ 1 \end{bmatrix} = \begin{bmatrix} 2 & 1 \\ 1 & 1 \end{bmatrix} \cdot \begin{bmatrix} \alpha \\ \beta \end{bmatrix} \qquad\qquad \text{(B.28)}$$

$$\vec{a} = \begin{bmatrix} 3 \\ 1 \end{bmatrix} \quad \mathbf{B} = \begin{bmatrix} 2 & 1 \\ 1 & 1 \end{bmatrix} \quad \vec{c} = \begin{bmatrix} \alpha \\ \beta \end{bmatrix} \quad \mathbf{B}^{-1} = \begin{bmatrix} 1 & -1 \\ -1 & 2 \end{bmatrix}$$

Using Eq. B.27 we obtain the solution $\vec{c} = [2 \quad -1]^T$.

For this particular problem it might seem to be faster to do it by hand, as above, instead of using Eq. B.27. This might also be true for such a simple problem, but in general using Eq. B.27 is definitely more efficient. Recall that you just have to define the matrix and vectors, then the computer solves them for you—independent of the number of equations and unknowns.

B.8 Similar Triangles

In Fig. B.4 two triangles are present. The outer triangle defined by the three points ABC and the inner triangle defined by the three points DBE. If the two triangles have the same angles, i.e., $\theta_1 = \theta_4$, $\theta_3 = \theta_5$, and $\theta_2 = \theta_2$, then the triangles are said to be *equiangular* or *similar*.

Fig. B.4 Two similar triangles, i.e., triangles with the same angles

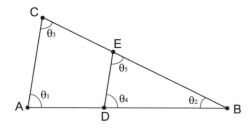

If we look at the outer triangle, then we know from trigonometry that

$$\frac{\|\overrightarrow{BC}\|}{\sin(\theta_1)} = \frac{\|\overrightarrow{CA}\|}{\sin(\theta_2)} = \frac{\|\overrightarrow{AB}\|}{\sin(\theta_3)} \tag{B.29}$$

For the inner triangle we have

$$\frac{\|\overrightarrow{BE}\|}{\sin(\theta_4)} = \frac{\|\overrightarrow{ED}\|}{\sin(\theta_2)} = \frac{\|\overrightarrow{DB}\|}{\sin(\theta_5)} \tag{B.30}$$

Combining the two equations we get the following relationships between the two triangles:

$$\frac{\sin(\theta_1)}{\sin(\theta_2)} = \frac{\sin(\theta_4)}{\sin(\theta_2)} = \frac{\|\overrightarrow{BC}\|}{\|\overrightarrow{CA}\|} = \frac{\|\overrightarrow{BE}\|}{\|\overrightarrow{ED}\|} \tag{B.31}$$

$$\frac{\sin(\theta_1)}{\sin(\theta_3)} = \frac{\sin(\theta_4)}{\sin(\theta_5)} = \frac{\|\overrightarrow{BC}\|}{\|\overrightarrow{AB}\|} = \frac{\|\overrightarrow{BE}\|}{\|\overrightarrow{DB}\|} \tag{B.32}$$

$$\frac{\sin(\theta_2)}{\sin(\theta_3)} = \frac{\sin(\theta_2)}{\sin(\theta_5)} = \frac{\|\overrightarrow{CA}\|}{\|\overrightarrow{AB}\|} = \frac{\|\overrightarrow{ED}\|}{\|\overrightarrow{DB}\|} \tag{B.33}$$

$$\frac{\|\overrightarrow{BC}\|}{\|\overrightarrow{AB}\|} = \frac{\|\overrightarrow{BE}\|}{\|\overrightarrow{DB}\|} \Leftrightarrow \frac{\|\overrightarrow{DB}\|}{\|\overrightarrow{AB}\|} = \frac{\|\overrightarrow{BE}\|}{\|\overrightarrow{BC}\|} \tag{B.34}$$

$$\frac{\|\overrightarrow{DB}\|}{\|\overrightarrow{AB}\|} = \frac{\|\overrightarrow{BE}\|}{\|\overrightarrow{BC}\|} \Leftrightarrow \frac{\|\overrightarrow{DB}\|}{\|\overrightarrow{AD}\| + \|\overrightarrow{DB}\|} = \frac{\|\overrightarrow{BE}\|}{\|\overrightarrow{BE}\| + \|\overrightarrow{EC}\|} \Leftrightarrow$$

$$\frac{\|\overrightarrow{DB}\|}{\|\overrightarrow{AD}\|} + 1 = 1 + \frac{\|\overrightarrow{BE}\|}{\|\overrightarrow{EC}\|} \Leftrightarrow \frac{\|\overrightarrow{DB}\|}{\|\overrightarrow{AD}\|} = \frac{\|\overrightarrow{BE}\|}{\|\overrightarrow{EC}\|} \tag{B.35}$$

$$\frac{\|\overrightarrow{BC}\|}{\|\overrightarrow{AB}\|} = \frac{\|\overrightarrow{BE}\|}{\|\overrightarrow{DB}\|} \Leftrightarrow \frac{\|\overrightarrow{BC}\|}{\|\overrightarrow{AB}\|} = \frac{\|\overrightarrow{EC}\|}{\|\overrightarrow{AD}\|} \Leftrightarrow \frac{\|\overrightarrow{AD}\|}{\|\overrightarrow{AB}\|} = \frac{\|\overrightarrow{EC}\|}{\|\overrightarrow{BC}\|} \tag{B.36}$$

References

1. J.K. Bowmaker, H.J.A. Dartnall, Visual pigments of rods and cones in a human retina. J. Physiol. **298**, 501–511 (1980)
2. I.L. Dryden, K. Mardia *Statistical Shape Analysis*, (Wiley, Chichester, 1998), pp. 347
3. R.C. Gonzalez, R.E. Woods, *Digital Image Processing*, 3 edn. (Prentice Hall, 2008)
4. E. Haber, J. Modersitzki, A multilevel method for image registration. SIAM J. Sci. Comput. **27**(5), 1594–1607 (2006)
5. T.B Moeslund, *Introduction to video and image processing: Building real systems and applications*, (Springer Science & Business Media, 2012)
6. W. Niblack, *An Introduction to Digital Image Processing*, (Prentice-Hall International, 1986)
7. N. Otsu, A threshold selection method from gray-level histograms. Automatica **11**, 285–296 (1975)
8. P.H. Schönemann, A generalized solution of the orthogonal Procrustes problem. Psychometrika **31**(1), 1–10 (1966)

© Springer Nature Switzerland AG 2020
R. R. Paulsen and T. B. Moeslund, *Introduction to Medical Image Analysis*,
Undergraduate Topics in Computer Science,
https://doi.org/10.1007/978-3-030-39364-9

Index

© Springer Nature Switzerland AG 2020
R. R. Paulsen and T. B. Moeslund, *Introduction to Medical Image Analysis*,
Undergraduate Topics in Computer Science,
https://doi.org/10.1007/978-3-030-39364-9

Printed in the United States
By Bookmasters